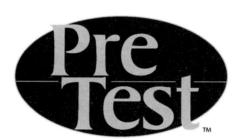

Neurology

PreTest™ Self-Assessment and Review

Notice

Medicine is an ever-changing science. As new research and clinical experience broaden our knowledge, changes in treatment and drug therapy are required. The authors and the publisher of this work have checked with sources believed to be reliable in their efforts to provide information that is complete and generally in accord with the standards accepted at the time of publication. However, in view of the possibility of human error or changes in medical sciences, neither the authors nor the publisher nor any other party who has been involved in the preparation or publication of this work warrants that the information contained herein is in every respect accurate or complete, and they disclaim all responsibility for any errors or omissions or for the results obtained from use of the information contained in this work. Readers are encouraged to confirm the information contained herein with other sources. For example and in particular, readers are advised to check the product information sheet included in the package of each drug they plan to administer to be certain that the information contained in this work is accurate and that changes have not been made in the recommended dose or in the contraindications for administration. This recommendation is of particular importance in connection with new or infrequently used drugs.

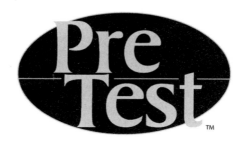

Neurology

PreTest™ Self-Assessment and Review
Sixth Edition

David J. Anschel, M.D.
Director of Adult Epilepsy Program, Long Island Comprehensive Epilepsy Center
Director of Intraoperative Neurophysiology, Stony Brook University Hospital
Assistant Professor of Neurology, SUNY at Stony Brook, NY
Associate Scientist, Brookhaven National Laboratory, Upton, NY

McGraw-Hill
Medical Publishing Division
New York   Chicago   San Francisco   Lisbon   London   Madrid   Mexico City
Milan   New Delhi   San Juan   Seoul   Singapore   Sydney   Toronto

The McGraw·Hill Companies

Neurology: PreTest™ Self-Assessment and Review, Sixth Edition

Copyright © 2006 by The McGraw-Hill Companies, Inc. All rights reserved. Printed in the United States of America. Except as permitted under the United States Copyright Act of 1976, no part of this publication may be reproduced or distributed in any form or by any means, or stored in a data base or retrieval system, without the prior written permission of the publisher.

PreTest is a trademark of The McGraw-Hill Companies, Inc.

3 4 5 6 7 8 9 0   DOC/DOC   0 9 8 7

ISBN 0-07-145550-7

This book was set in Berkeley by North Market Street Graphics.
The editor was Catherine A. Johnson.
The production supervisor was Sherri Souffrance.
Project management was provided by North Market Street Graphics.
The cover designer was Mary McKeon.
RR Donnelley was printer and binder.

This book is printed on acid-free paper.

Library of Congress Cataloging-in-Publication Data

Anschel, David.
    Neurology : PreTest self-assessment and review. / David J. Anschel.—6th ed.
      p. ; cm.
    Includes bibliographical references and index.
    ISBN 0-07-145550-7
      1. Neurology—Examinations, questions, etc.   2. Neurology—Outlines, syllabi, etc.
    I. Title.
    [DNLM: 1. Nervous System Diseases—Examination Questions. WL 18.2 A617n 2006]
    RC343.5.A57 2006
    616.80076—dc22   2005056248

Student Reviewers

Bobby Armin
UCLA School of Medicine
Class of 2005

Suzanne Crandall
College of Osteopathic Medicine
Kansas City University School of Medicine and Biosciences
Class of 2005

Kevin L. Olson
Medical College of Virginia
Class of 2005

Contents

Nutritional and Metabolic Disorders

Dementia and Cognitive Disorders

Movement Disorders

Disorders of Myelination

Developmental and Hereditary Disorders

Neuromuscular Disorders

Toxic Injuries

Eye Disease and Visual Disturbances

Introduction

Neurology: PreTest™ Self-Assessment and Review, Sixth Edition, is intended to provide medical students, as well as house officers and physicians, with a convenient tool for assessing and improving their knowledge of neurology. The 500 questions in this book are similar in format and complexity to those included in Step 2 of the United States Medical Licensing Examination (USMLE). They may also be a useful study tool for Step 3 and clerkship examinations.

Each question in this book has a corresponding answer, a reference to a text that provides background for the answer, and a short discussion of various issues raised by the question and its answer. A listing of references for the entire book follows the last chapter.

To simulate the time constraints imposed by the qualifying examinations for which this book is intended as a practice guide, the student or physician should allot about one minute for each question. After answering all questions in a chapter, as much time as necessary should be spent reviewing the explanations for each question at the end of the chapter. Attention should be given to all explanations, even if the examinee answered the question correctly. Those seeking more information on a subject should refer to the reference materials listed or to other standard texts in neurology.

The Neurological Examination and Diagnostic Tests

Questions

DIRECTIONS: Each item below contains a question followed by suggested responses. Select the **one best** response to each question.

1. An 85-year-old man is being evaluated for gait difficulties. On examination it is found that joint proprioception is absent in his toes. People with impaired position sense will usually fall if they stand with their feet together and do which of the following?

a.   Flex the neck
b.   Extend their arms in front of them
c.   Flex the knees
d.   Turn the head
e.   Close their eyes

2. A 42-year-old man notices that his right pupil is smaller than the left. His wife has also commented that the right eye is "droopy looking." The only remarkable recent history is that he was tackled a little hard while playing football the day before. Magnetic resonance imaging (MRI) of the head and neck in this patient would be expected to show which of the following?

a.   Increased T2 signal in a periventricular distribution
b.   Contrast enhancement along the tentorial margin
c.   Increased T1 signal in the wall of the left carotid artery
d.   Enlarged optic nerve in the orbit
e.   Thrombosed cavernous sinus aneurysm

3. A 21-year-old woman presents with right arm loss of sensation that has been progressive over a few days. Her physician orders an MRI, which is pictured below. Which of the following is the most likely process?

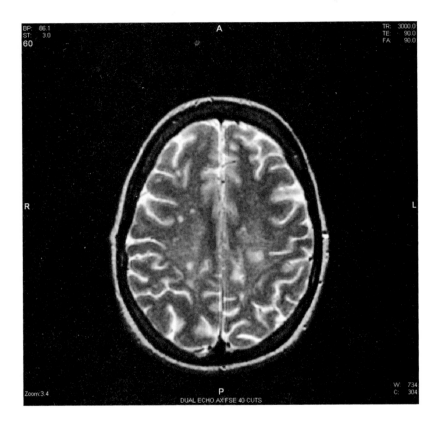

a. Ischemic
b. Demyelinating
c. Neoplastic
d. Hemorrhagic
e. Psychogenic

4. A 62-year-old right-handed man has "involuntary twitches" of his left hand. He first noticed between 6 months and 1 year ago that when he is at rest, his left hand shakes. He can stop the shaking by looking at his hand and concentrating. The shaking does not impair his activities in any way. He has no trouble holding a glass of water. There is no tremor in his right hand and the lower extremities are not affected. He has had no trouble walking. There have been no behavioral or language changes. On examination, a left hand tremor is evident when he is distracted. Handwriting is mildly tremulous. He is very mildly bradykinetic on the left. The most likely exam finding would be which of the following?

a. Upper motor neuron pattern of weakness on the left
b. Lower motor neuron pattern of weakness on the left
c. Bilateral upper motor neuron pattern of weakness
d. Mild cogwheel rigidity on the left only with distraction
e. Bilateral severe cogwheel rigidity

5. Tremor in the hands that is most obvious when the patient is awake and trying to perform an action is most likely due to disease in which of the following structures?

a. Thalamus
b. Cerebellum
c. Substantia nigra
d. Spinal cord
e. Internal capsule

6. In the person with Parkinson's disease, the tremor that is evident when a limb is at rest changes in what way when the patient falls asleep?

a. It becomes more rapid
b. Its amplitude increases
c. It generalizes to limbs that were uninvolved when the patient was awake
d. It disappears
e. It transforms into choreiform movements

7. A 25-year-old woman with a history of epilepsy presents to the emergency room with impaired attention and unsteadiness of gait. Her phenytoin level is 37. She has white blood cells in her urine and has a mildly elevated TSH. Examination of the eyes would be most likely to show which of the following?

a. Weakness of abduction of the left eye
b. Lateral beating movements of the eyes
c. Impaired convergence
d. Papilledema
e. Impaired upward gaze

8. A 75-year-old generally healthy man has noticed worsening problems maneuvering over the past 4 months. He has particular trouble getting out of low seats and off toilets. He most likely has which of the following?

a. Poor fine finger movements
b. Poor rapid alternating movements
c. Distal muscle weakness
d. Proximal muscle weakness
e. Gait apraxia

9. A 50-year-old right-handed man has presented to a neurologist because of gradually progressive hearing loss. A vibrating tuning fork is applied to the center of his forehead. This helps to establish which of the following?

a. Which ear has the wider range of frequency perception
b. Which ear has the larger external auditory meatus
c. Which ear has infection of the external ear canal
d. Which ear has the longer eustachian tube
e. Which ear has conductive or sensorineural hearing loss

10. A 38-year-old woman says that she is "dizzy." A more careful history reveals that she has an abnormal sensation of movement intermittently. Examination reveals horizontal rhythmic eye movements on leftward gaze. A T1 MRI image from this patient is shown. Electronystagmography is most likely to support which of the following diagnoses?

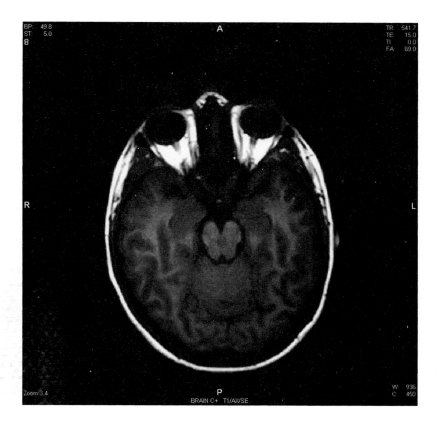

a. Ocular bobbing
b. Pontine hemorrhage
c. Cervicomedullary junction glioma
d. Episodic vertigo
e. Brainstem stroke

11. A 48-year-old left-handed man develops increased sensitivity to sound in his left ear. A brain MRI reveals a posterior fossa mass. This symptom may develop in one ear with damage to which of the following ipsilateral cranial nerves?

a. V
b. VII
c. VIII
d. IX
e. X

12. A 42-year-old woman is being evaluated for gait difficulties. On examination, it is found that her ability to walk along a straight line touching the heel of one foot to the toe of the other is impaired. This finding is most common with which of the following?

a. Cerebellar dysfunction
b. Parietal lobe damage
c. Temporal lobe damage
d. Ocular motor disturbances
e. Dysesthesias in the feet

13. A 55-year-old woman is being examined. The clinician notices the presence of fine twitching movements beneath the surface of the tongue and wasting of one side of the tongue. This finding suggests damage to which of the following cranial nerves?

a. V
b. VII
c. IX
d. X
e. XII

14. A 46-year-old longshoreman has lower back pain radiating down the posterior aspect of his left leg, and paresthesias in the lateral aspect of his left foot. This has been present for 6 months. Strength and bowel and bladder function have been normal. Examination would be most likely to show which of the following?

a. Left Babinski sign
b. Loss of pinprick sensation over the web space between the first and second digits of the left foot
c. Hyperreflexia at the left knee jerk
d. Hyporeflexia in the left Achilles tendon reflex
e. Decreased rectal tone

15. A 28-year-old graduate student presents with confusion and mild right hemiparesis developing over the course of an evening. His girlfriend relates that he has been having severe headaches each morning for the past 2 weeks. While being evaluated in the emergency room, he has a generalized tonic-clonic seizure. When examined 2 h later, he is lethargic and unable to recall recent events, has difficulty naming, and has a right pronator drift. There is mild weakness of abduction of the eyes bilaterally. Funduscopic examination might be expected to show which of the following?

a. Pigmentary degeneration of the retina
b. Hollenhorst plaques
c. Retinal venous pulsations
d. Blurring of the margins of the optic disc
e. Pallor of the optic disc

16. Taking a normal, awake person who is lying supine with head slightly elevated (30°) and irrigating one external auditory meatus with warm water will induce which of the following?

a. Tonic deviation of the eyes toward the ear that is stimulated
b. Nystagmus in both eyes toward the ear that is stimulated
c. Tonic deviation of the ipsilateral eye toward the ear that is stimulated
d. Nystagmus in both eyes away from the ear that is stimulated
e. Tonic deviation of both eyes away from the ear that is stimulated

17. A 33-year-old woman has the acute onset of right orbital pain after a tennis match. The following morning, her 10-year-old son comments that her right eye looks funny. On examination, she has a mild right ptosis and anisocoria. The right pupil is 2 mm smaller than the left, but both react normally to direct light stimulation. Visual acuity, visual fields, and eye movements are normal. The site of injury is due to interruption of fibers from which of the following structures?

a. Optic tract
b. Optic chiasm
c. Cranial nerve III
d. T1 nerve root
e. Superior cervical ganglion

18. An 81-year-old woman with a history of type 2 diabetes mellitus and atrial fibrillation presents with right body weakness and slurred speech. She realized that there was a problem on awakening in the morning, and her husband called EMS, who brought her to the emergency room. There are no word-finding difficulties, dysesthesia, or headaches. She is taking warfarin. Physical exam findings include blood pressure of 210/95 and irregularly irregular heartbeat. There is left-side neglect with slurred speech. There is a corticospinal pattern of weakness of the right body, with the face and upper extremity worse than the lower extremity. Routine chemistries and cell counts are normal. Her INR is 1.7. A head CT reveals a large right-sided subdural hematoma. The intracranial material appearing most dense on computed tomography (CT) of the head is which of the following?

a. Blood clot
b. White matter
c. Gray matter
d. Cerebrospinal fluid (CSF)
e. Pia mater

19. A 15-year-old boy developed a left Bell's palsy over the course of 1 week. He was treated with acyclovir and prednisone. Over the next 3 months he seemed to recover almost fully. However, he has noticed involuntary twitching at the left corner of the mouth each time he tries to blink the left eye. This is most likely caused by which of the following?

a. A habit spasm
b. Cerebellar damage producing impaired coordination
c. Aberrant regeneration of the facial nerve
d. Trigeminal neuralgia
e. Focal seizures

20. You are working in the emergency room when a 30-year-old man presents with a headache that started yesterday. As he was shoveling snow, he felt a sudden pain in the front of his head. The pain does not throb and has been relatively constant since. He says that now his neck also has become a little stiff. He carries a diagnosis of migraine headaches, but says that this is different than his usual headaches. He is afebrile and has a normal exam except for slight photophobia and mild discomfort with neck flexion. Which of the following is the most appropriate next step in management?

a. Obtain a brain MRI
b. Obtain a brain CT
c. Obtain a cerebral angiogram
d. Obtain an EEG
e. Obtain a psychiatry consult

21. A 56-year-old right-handed woman presents to the emergency room with a sudden-onset, severe, left-sided headache. The pain began when she stood up from her couch while watching TV. A head CT is normal. Which of the following is the most appropriate next step in management of this patient?

a. Begin intravenous heparin
b. Perform a lumbar puncture
c. Obtain a brain MRI
d. Obtain a cerebral angiogram
e. Give the patient a prescription for zolmitriptan and send her home

22. A 60-year-old man is clinically suspected to have had a subarachnoid hemorrhage. A lumbar puncture shows 7000 red blood cells in tube 1 and 7200 in tube 4. There are 9 white blood cells in each. The fluid is xanthochromic. The opening pressure is 22 cm H_2O. Which of the following is the best next step in managing this case?

a. Arrange for a cerebral angiogram and call a neurosurgical consult
b. Give the patient a prescription for sumatriptan and send him home
c. Immediately give 2 g of intravenous ceftriaxone
d. Immediately start intravenous acyclovir
e. Repeat the lumbar puncture

23. A 28-year-old man presents to the emergency room with a severe headache. It is different than any that he has ever had before. It is in the right posterior region and not throbbing. The headache started suddenly, about 5 h ago, while he was watching television and eating pizza. He is now noticing some mild neck stiffness and blurry vision. Examination is significant for weakness of abduction of the right eye. Which of the following is the most definitive test for identifying intracranial aneurysms?

a. MRI scanning
b. CT scanning
c. Single photon emission computed tomography (SPECT)
d. Positron emission tomography (PET)
e. Cerebral angiography

24. In this MRI scan, the site most likely to produce a noncommunicating hydrocephalus when it is obstructed is identified by which of the following?

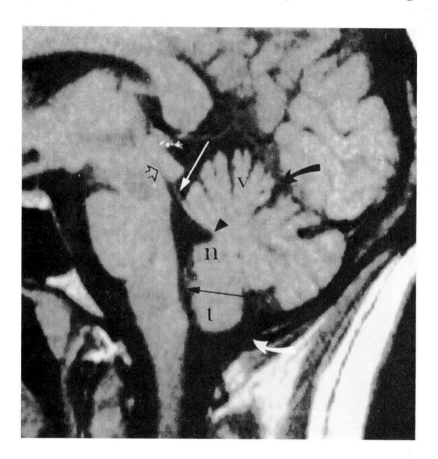

a. Open black arrow
b. Straight white arrow
c. Curved black arrow
d. Black arrowhead
e. Straight black arrow

25. The location of the cerebellar tonsil in the MRI scan suggests which of the following?

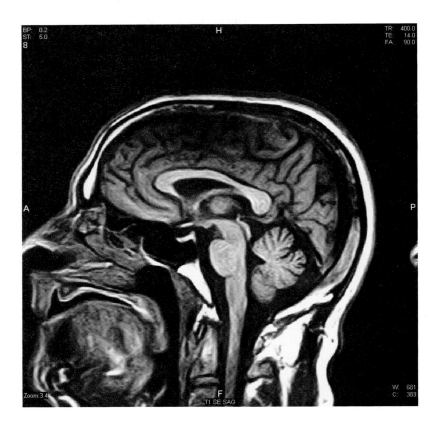

a. Arnold-Chiari type 1 malformation
b. Arnold-Chiari type 2 malformation
c. Giant cisterna magna
d. Dandy-Walker syndrome
e. Normal posterior fossa

26. A 46 year-old woman with depression has a brain CT performed at the request of her psychiatrist. There is the incidental finding of a dense mass that appears to originate from the tentorium cerebelli. The tentorium cerebelli separates the superior cerebellum from the cerebrum and is a common site of origin for which of the following?

a. Meningiomas
b. Ependymomas
c. Hemangioblastomas
d. Medulloblastomas
e. Astrocytomas

27. A 35-year-old woman has noticed that over the past 3 to 5 months she has had some difficulties with balance, particularly when she closes her eyes. On examination, she has decreased hearing in her left ear and also left body dysdiadochokinesia. Her physician orders a head CT. Given this CT scan, which was obtained without contrast enhancement, the physician must assume that the posterior fossa mass at the arrow is which of the following?

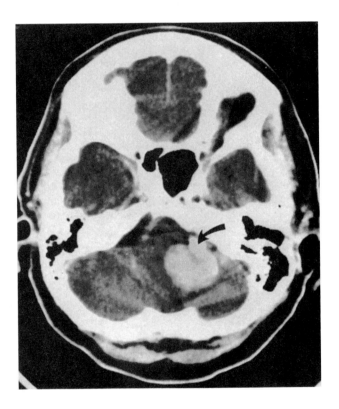

a. Normal
b. Calcified
c. Highly vascular
d. Granulomatous
e. Highly cystic

28. A 35-year-old woman presents with slowly evolving left arm ataxia, left-sided head tilt, dysarthria, and left facial weakness. The patient denies vertigo, tinnitus, or hearing loss. MRI reveals a posterior fossa mass that lies close to the bone and enhances with contrast. Which of the following is the most likely explanation for this lesion?

a. Cerebellar infarction
b. Cerebellar hemorrhage
c. Meningioma
d. Schwannoma
e. Astrocytoma

29. Which of the following is the most appropriate course of action for the management of most meningiomas?

a. Anticoagulation
b. Triple therapy with isoniazid, rifampin, and ethambutol
c. Surgical resection
d. Proton beam irradiation
e. Craniospinal axis irradiation

30. A patient with bilateral posterior fossa masses has café au lait spots and reports a family history of bilateral hearing loss at a relatively young age. A gene abnormality should be suspected on which chromosome?

a. 5
b. 13
c. 17
d. 21
e. 22

31. A 65-year-old diabetic man has a history of a cerebellar stroke. The stroke occurred 5 years ago, and he says that he has now fully recovered. He cannot recall the symptoms, but his medical records state that he presented with left-sided dysdiadochokinesia. Dysdiadochokinesia is an impairment of which of the following?

a. Successive finger movements
b. Heel-to-toe walking
c. Rapid alternating movements
d. Tremor suppression
e. Conjugate eye movements

32. A 27-year-old normal woman is having a routine EEG examination. The study begins with a 5-min recording of her sleeping. Then she is awakened and given photic stimulation. Next she is alert and awake, lying with her eyes closed in a quiet room. At this point she will exhibit what frequency of EEG activity over the occipital and parietal areas bilaterally?

a. 0 to 3 Hz
b. 4 to 7 Hz
c. 8 to 13 Hz
d. 14 to 25 Hz
e. 26 to 45 Hz

33. Below is shown a T1-weighted postcontrast brain MRI of a 58-year-old woman. The abnormality is due to a glioblastoma multiforme. Which of the following was most likely to be her presenting symptom?

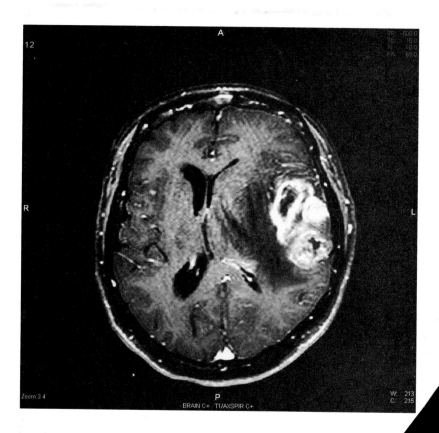

a. Aphasia
b. Neglect
c. Left hemiparesis
d. Left homonymous hemianopia
e. Alexia without agraphia

DIRECTIONS: Each group of questions below consists of lettered options followed by a set of numbered items. For each numbered item, select the **one** lettered option with which it is **most** closely associated. Each lettered option may be used once, more than once, or not at all.

Questions 34–38

For each clinical scenario, choose the single study that is most likely to establish the diagnosis and direct further treatment.

a. MRI of the brain
b. Brain biopsy
c. Nerve conduction (NC) studies
d. CSF analysis
e. EEG
f. Serum creatine phosphokinase (CPK)
g. Cerebral angiography
h. Myelography of the spinal canal
i. Cranial computerized axial tomography (CAT)
j. Skull x-ray
k. Visual evoked responses (VER)
l. Nerve biopsy

34. A 65-year-old man with a history of atrial fibrillation is brought into the emergency room at 1:00 P.M. because of the acute onset of right-sided weakness and inability to speak beginning at noon. On examination, he is alert but unable to speak. He follows simple one-step commands. There is left gaze deviation and impaired rightward gaze. Flaccid paresis of the right face and arm is present, but he is able to lift his right leg off the bed. ⸱ are decreased on the right side.

⸱ₒss woman is admitted to the hospital with ulcer-
ₒf burning in her feet and lower legs, but
'⸱n is ulcerated. She is unable to
gether. Her deep tendon reflexes
esting of her strength and sensa-
ₒion sense are evident in her hands
siflexion of the ankles and wrists.

36. A 7-year-old boy has recurrent staring episodes while at school. His school performance is poor. The episodes never last more than 30 s, and afterward he immediately resumes normal attention. There are no lip-smacking movements or other automatisms. He never falls down during the episodes. If he is walking or eating during the episode, he merely stops. He is unaware of this behavior.

37. A previously healthy 7-month-old infant is brought to the ER after having had three generalized convulsions. The infant has a stiff neck, is poorly responsive to the examiner, and has a rectal temperature of 38.9°C (102°F). The parents report that 1 day of diarrhea preceded this episode.

38. A 70-year-old right-handed woman with a history of polio describes 1 month of increasing difficulty rising from a chair and walking. She also has trouble combing her hair and cooking, and there is mild swallowing trouble, but only with solids. Her legs and upper arms are painful and mildly swollen. Periungual telangiectasias are seen. ESR is 61.

Questions 39–45

For each clinical scenario, choose the CSF pattern most likely to be found.

	Protein Content (mg/dL)	Glucose Content (mg/dL)	WBC (per µL)	RBC (per µL)	Opening Pressure (mmH$_2$O)	Gamma Globulin Appearance	% Protein
Normal values	15–45	40–70	0–5	0	100–180	Clear	3–12
a.	40	75	3	0	430	Clear	8
b.	300	86	7	0	120	Yellow	12
c.	65	80	8	0	110	Clear	17
d.	95	12	150	3	200	Milky	13
e.	120	65	85	15	300	Cloudy	15
f.	45	78	3	0	130	Clear	7
g.	250	68	20	9808	190	Yellow	14

39. A 26-year-old woman with a 7-year history of epilepsy develops a generalized convulsion while shopping. She is taken to an ER, but no one accompanying her is aware of the previous history of epilepsy. Because she has a protracted postictal period, numerous investigations are performed over the course of the next hour. CT scan is completely normal, but her arterial blood gases reveal a mild acidosis.

40. A 72-year-old man is brought to the ER in a coma. He has a fever and was observed to have a generalized tonic-clonic seizure just prior to arriving in the ER. His family reports that he had lethargy and cough about 1 week prior to the acute deterioration. On the day of his seizure, he developed a headache and blurred vision. He had some vomiting early in the day and became more stuporous as the day progressed. There is no evidence of alcohol or drug use.

41. A 19-year-old man notices discomfort in his ankles within a few days of recovering from an upper respiratory infection. Over the next 7 days, he develops progressive weakness in both of his legs and subsequently in his arms. He has no loss of sensation in his limbs, despite the progressive loss of strength. He does not lose bladder or bowel control, but on the tenth day of his weakness he develops problems with breathing and requires ventilatory assistance.

42. A 40-year-old man was involved in an automobile accident. There is an obvious laceration on his head, and he has neck pain. Police at the scene report that he was unconscious when they arrived, but the patient cannot recall this loss of consciousness. In fact, he cannot remember the accident or events within 10 min prior to the accident. On examination, he has obvious neck stiffness and photophobia. Within a few hours of his arrival at the ER, he develops vomiting. Lumbar puncture is delayed until after an MRI can be obtained. The tap is performed 2 days after the accident because the patient is still confused and irritable.

43. A 22-year-old woman is brought to the hospital in a coma. She has had changes in her behavior characterized by excessive suspiciousness and facetiousness over the month prior to her hospitalization. One week prior to her hospitalization, she had visual and auditory hallucinations. Drug testing reveals no apparent illicit drug use. On the day of admission, she had a generalized seizure and lapsed into a coma. MRI shows unilateral changes in the temporal lobe.

44. A 26-year-old man develops bed wetting and transient sexual dysfunction that resolves over the course of 6 weeks. One month later, he notices a pins-and-needles sensation in his right leg that never clears completely. On examination, he has hyperreflexia in both of his legs and past-pointing in his right arm. His gait is slightly ataxic, and he is unable to perform tandem gait.

45. A 26-year-old woman weighing in excess of 300 lb complains of headache and blurred vision that began 2 weeks prior to consulting a physician. She has no vomiting or diplopia. Examination of her eyes reveals florid papilledema but without hemorrhages. Her neurologic examination is otherwise entirely normal. She had a similar problem while pregnant with her fourth child.

The Neurological Examination and Diagnostic Tests

Answers

1. The answer is e. (*Victor, pp 123, 165–166.*) Standing with the feet together and the eyes closed is the Romberg test. The person with poor position sense needs visual cues to remain standing. This test was introduced as a helpful way to check for deficits associated with tabes dorsalis, a form of neurosyphilis. In tabes dorsalis, the dorsal columns of the spinal cord are damaged. These dorsal or posterior columns carry the nerve fibers that transmit vibration and position sense to the brain. With the widespread use of penicillin, tabes dorsalis has become rare in industrialized nations, and impaired position sense is much more likely to be a consequence of diabetes mellitus or alcoholism. In both of these conditions, the impaired position sense is much more likely to be a consequence of damage to nerves in the limbs than of damage to the posterior columns of the spinal cord. In performing the test, it is important to remember that even normal people will tend to sway slightly more when their eyes are closed, and that those with loss of cerebellar function will also sway more with loss of visual cues.

2. The answer is c. (*Greenberg, pp 693–694.*) The most likely cause of this patient's symptoms and signs is a carotid dissection. Dissections are caused by a tear in the intimal lining of the vessel with penetration of blood beneath the intimal surface, forming an intramural hematoma (blood clot within the wall of the vessel). This may be seen as an area of increased signal within the lining of the vessel on T1-weighted images, on which a blood clot appears bright. Typically, this takes a crescentic pattern, and the lumen of the vessel is displaced eccentrically. An increased T2 signal in a periventricular distribution is typical of the plaques of demyelinating disease seen in multiple sclerosis. Contrast enhancement along the tentorial margin might be seen in inflammatory diseases of the dura mater or meninges. An enlarged optic nerve might be seen in the setting of optic neuritis or infiltration of the nerve by a tumor or other process, and this would be expected to cause visual impairment. A cavernous sinus aneurysm that is sufficient to produce oculosympathetic palsy would be expected to cause other deficits in ocular motility, because the cranial nerves subserving oculomotor function course through the cavernous sinus.

3. The answer is b. (*Victor, pp 954–977.*) The history and MRI are consistent with a demyelinating process, such as acute disseminated encephalomyelitis (ADEM) or multiple sclerosis. The MRI shown is a T2-weighted image. Several areas of abnormal high signal are apparent. Magnetic resonance imaging depends primarily upon the water content of tissues, but it can be customized to look at more specific properties of tissues. A variety of methods are available for affecting the information produced by and analyzing the information generated by MRI. The T2-weighted image is not specific for demyelination, but it is useful in following changes in plaques of demyelination, an application that has been used in studies of agents useful in the management of multiple sclerosis.

4. The answer is d. (*Victor, pp 1128–1132.*) This patient gives a typical history for early Parkinson's disease. The classic triad is asymmetric resting tremor, rigidity, and bradykinesia. The rigidity is generally severe later, not early in the disease. Parkinson's disease is not characterized by weakness.

5. The answer is b. (*Victor, p 90.*) Intention or kinetic tremors are most characteristic of damage to the cerebellum. Kinetic tremors of the hand or arms are most common with disease of the cerebellar hemispheres, but they may also develop with damage to the spinocerebellar tracts of the spinal cord. Damage to the substantia nigra, such as that occurring in Parkinson's disease, produces a resting tremor that abates when the patient moves the involved limb intentionally. Damage to the thalamus is more likely to produce a sensory disturbance. Tremors may develop with spinal cord damage, but they do not follow a typical pattern and do not suggest a spinal cord origin.

6. The answer is d. (*Watts and Koller, p 235.*) Patients with Parkinson's disease often have a characteristic pill-rolling tremor of the hand while they are awake. The tremors associated with Parkinson's disease are worse when the patient is at rest and not moving the affected limb. Paradoxically, this resting tremor ceases when relaxation progresses to sleep. In fact, most tremors and other types of movement disorders caused by disease of the caudate, putamen, and globus pallidus (i.e., the basal ganglia) and of the substantia nigra remit during sleep. Choreiform movements are jumping or dancelike movements and occur with Wilson's disease (hepatolenticular degeneration) and Huntington's disease, a hereditary degenerative disease of the basal ganglia.

7. The answer is b. (*Victor, pp 290–293.*) Most rhythmic to-and-fro movements of the eyes are called *nystagmus*. Nystagmus has a fast component in one direction and a slow component in the opposite direction. Nystagmus with a fast component to the right is called *right-beating* nystagmus. Phenytoin (Dilantin) may evoke nystagmus at levels of 20 to 30 mg/dL. The eye movements typically appear as a laterally beating nystagmus on gaze to either side; this type of nystagmus is called *gaze-evoked*. If the patient has nystagmus on looking directly forward, he or she is said to have nystagmus in the position of *primary gaze*. Therapeutic levels for phenytoin are usually 10 to 20 mg/dL, and some patients develop asymptomatic nystagmus even within that range. Ataxia, dysarthria, impaired judgment, and lethargy may also occur at toxic levels of phenytoin. Many other drugs, such as alcohol, barbiturates, and other sedatives, also evoke nystagmus. Weakness of abduction of the left eye, or *abducens palsy*, is due either to injury to the sixth cranial nerve or to increased intracranial pressure. Impaired convergence can occur normally with age or may be a sign of injury to the midbrain. Papilledema is a sign of increased intracranial pressure. Impaired upward gaze may occur in many conditions, but would not be expected to occur due to a toxic phenytoin level.

8. The answer is d. (*Kasper, p 2540.*) With primary muscle diseases, such as polymyositis, weakness usually develops in proximal muscle groups much more than in distal groups. This means that weakness will be most obvious in the hip girdle and shoulder girdle muscles. The hip girdle is usually affected before the shoulder girdle. To get out of a low seat, the affected person may need to pull him- or herself up using both arms. Persons with more generalized weakness or problems with coordination are less likely to report problems with standing from a seated position. Poor rapid alternating movements and poor fine finger movements usually develop with impaired coordination, such as that due to cerebellar damage.

With severe weakness in the limbs, patients will do poorly on these tests of function as well. With proximal muscle weakness, the affected person will usually perform relatively well on these tests of distal limb coordination.

9. The answer is e. (*Victor, p 306.*) The vibrations from a tuning fork placed on top of the head are transmitted through the skull to both ears. Bone conduction of sound through the skull should be equal in both ears. With sensorineural hearing loss, the patient will hear the midline fork more loudly in the unaffected ear. Sensorineural hearing loss is the deafness that develops with injury to the receptor cells in the cochlea or to the cochlear division of the auditory nerve. In conductive hearing loss, the vibrations of the tuning fork are perceived as louder in the affected ear. With this type of hearing loss, the injury is in the system of membranes and ossicles designed to focus the sound on the cochlea. Impairment of the conductive system causes the vibrations of the tuning fork to be transmitted to the cochlea directly through the skull. Much like a person with cotton stuffed into the external auditory meati, the patient with the conductive hearing loss has impaired perception of sound coming from around him or her but an enhanced perception of his or her own voice. This type of tuning fork test is called the Weber test.

10. The answer is d. (*Victor, pp 290–292, 315–325.*) Abnormal patterns of eye movement may help localize disease in the central or peripheral nervous system in patients with vertigo. The retina is negatively charged in comparison with the cornea, which creates a dipole that may be monitored during electronystagmography studies with electrodes placed on the skin about the eyes. Movement of the most posterior elements of the retina toward an electrode is registered as a negative voltage change at that electrode. Damage to the pons may produce characteristic conjugate deviations of the eyes. The conjugate eye movements are rhythmic and directed downward, but they lack the rapid component characteristic of nystagmus. This type of abnormal eye movement is called *ocular bobbing*. A lesion at the cervicomedullary junction, such as a meningioma at the foramen magnum, will produce a down-beating nystagmus with both eyes rhythmically deviating downward, with the rapid component of this nystagmus directed downward as well. *Cervicomedullary* refers to the cervical spinal cord and the medulla oblongata. Damage to the midbrain, thalamus, or hypothalamus may disturb eye movements, but down-beating nystagmus would not ordinarily develop with damage to these structures. The pictured MRI is entirely normal.

11. The answer is b. (*Victor, pp 1451–1452.*) The facial nerve innervates the stapedius muscle of the middle ear. With paralysis of this muscle, undamped transmission of acoustic signals across the stapedius bone of the middle ear produces hyperacusis. Hyperacusis is an indication that the damage to the facial nerve is close to its origin from the brainstem, because the nerve to the stapedius muscle is one of the first branches of the facial nerve. The tensor tympani is controlled by the motor fibers in the fifth cranial nerve. With damage to this nerve, the tympanic membrane has some inappropriate slack, but the patient does not usually comment on increased sensitivity to sound in the affected ear.

12. The answer is a. (*DeMyer, pp 379–380.*) Walking along a straight line with the heel of one foot touching the toe of the other foot is called *heel-to-toe walking*, or *tandem gait*. It is a routine test for ethanol intoxication because alcohol exposure impairs the coordination of gait as governed by the cerebellum. Tandem gait will be abnormal with many other problems, including weakness, poor position sense, vertigo, and leg tremors, but such abnormality in the absence of these other problems suggests a cerebellar basis for the problem.

13. The answer is e. (*Victor, pp 1459–1460.*) The hypoglossal nerve innervates the tongue. The fine movements noted under the surface of the tongue with injury to the hypoglossal nerve are called *fasciculations* and are an indication of denervation. They are presumed to occur through hypersensitivity to acetylcholine acting at the denervated neuromuscular junction. Atrophy and fasciculations are likely to occur together and are highly suggestive of denervation of the tongue. This is most often seen with brainstem disease, such as stroke or bulbar amyotrophic lateral sclerosis (ALS), or with transection of the hypoglossal nerve.

14. The answer is d. (*Victor, pp 213–215.*) This patient has a history most consistent with a herniated lumbar disk. The most common locations for lumbar disk herniation are between the fifth lumbar and first sacral vertebrae (producing S1 nerve root compression) and between the fourth and fifth lumbar vertebrae (producing L5 root compression). S1 nerve root compression, or radiculopathy, is associated with pain in the lower back or buttock region, often radiating down the posterior thigh and calf to the lateral and plantar surfaces of the foot and affecting the fourth and fifth digits of the foot. Motor function of the foot and toe flexors, toe abductors, and hamstring muscles may be impaired, but more often it is not. Bowel and bladder function are usually preserved. The loss of the ankle jerk, or Achilles tendon reflex, is often the only objective sign of S1 radiculopathy. Deep tendon reflexes such as the ankle jerk are diminished or lost when there is damage to the sensory fibers from the tendon stretch organs.

A Babinski sign is an indication of upper motor neuron damage, which is not expected in this case with preserved autonomic and motor function. Loss of pinprick sensation over the web space between first and second toes is found in association with injury to the fifth lumbar nerve root or to the peroneal nerve. Hyperreflexia of the knee jerk is another sign of an upper motor neuron lesion and would not be expected in this case. Straight-leg raising (Lasègue maneuver) is used to determine whether symptoms are due to nerve root compression by stretching the nerve root. With compression, lifting the leg passively may be limited to between 20 and 30°. This test may be positive on the contralateral side (crossed straight-leg-raising sign), but it is usually more prominent on the affected side.

15. The answer is d. (*Victor, pp 258–260, 684–686.*) The presentation with subacute onset of morning headaches culminating in confusion, right hemiparesis, and seizure in a young person suggests an expanding mass lesion, most likely a tumor. The weakness of eye abduction bilaterally is what may be referred to as a false localizing sign. Although this suggests injury to the sixth cranial nerves bilaterally, the injury is not restricted to the sixth cranial nerve. The increase in intracranial pressure (ICP) from the mass causes stretching of the sixth-nerve fibers, which consequently leads to their dysfunction. Diplopia may be appreciated only on lateral gaze, which requires full function of the sixth nerve. Funduscopic exam in such a case would most likely reflect changes of increased ICP. The first sign of this is usually blurring of the margins of the optic disc and elevation of the disc due to swelling. Changes in the optic disc—the area in which all the nerve fibers from the retina come together and exit as the optic nerve— occur with problems other than increased ICP (such as optic neuritis), but blurring of the margins should be routinely considered a sign of increased ICP. This is especially true if the appearance of the disc has changed in association with the development of headache, obtundation, and vomiting. Pigmentary degeneration of the retina may occur with some infections, such as congenital toxoplasmosis or cytomegalovirus, or as part of a hereditary metabolic disorder, as in retinitis pigmentosa. Hollenhorst plaques are cholesterol and calcific deposits seen in the retinal arterioles in the setting of atheroembolism to the eye, along with visual loss. Retinal venous pulsations are typically not present when there is increased ICP, although they may also be absent in up to 15% of normal individuals.

16. The answer is b. *(Victor, p 319.)* Caloric stimulation of the ear drives the endolymphatic fluid in the inner ear up or down, depending on whether warm or cold water is used. By tilting the head of a supine patient up 30° from the horizontal, the semicircular canal responsible for detecting horizontal head movements is placed in a vertical plane, and caloric stimulation drives the endolymph in that canal more effectively than it will the endolymph in the other semicircular canals. The vestibular organ exposed to warm water sends impulses to the brainstem that indicate that the head is moving to the side that is being warmed. The eyes deviate to the opposite side to maintain fixation on their targets, but the eye movement actually breaks fixation. A reflex nystagmus toward the ear that is being stimulated develops as the brain tries to establish refixation while the vestibular signals repeatedly prompt deviation of the eyes contralateral to the warm stimulus.

17. The answer is e. *(Victor, p 319. Kandel, p 963.)* The presence of ptosis and miosis indicate oculosympathetic palsy, or Horner syndrome. This indicates injury to the sympathetic supply to the eye. This pathway begins in the hypothalamus, travels down through the lateral aspect of the brainstem, synapses in the intermediolateral cell column of the spinal cord, exits the spinal cord at the level of T1, and synapses again in the superior cervical ganglion. From there, postganglionic fibers travel along the surface of the common carotid and internal carotid artery until branches leave along the ophthalmic artery to the eye. Fibers of the sympathetic nervous system, which are destined to serve the sudomotor function of the forehead, travel with the external carotid artery. Thus, diseases affecting the internal carotid artery and the overlying sympathetic plexus do not produce anhidrosis, the third element of Horner syndrome. In this case, the occurrence of painful Horner syndrome acutely after vigorous activity is virtually diagnostic of carotid artery dissection. Dissections may occur more frequently in migraineurs.

The preservation of visual fields and acuity excludes significant disease of the optic tract and chiasm, which also would not be expected to cause ptosis. Lesions of cranial nerve (CN) III do cause ptosis, but they would also be expected to cause ipsilateral mydriasis, or pupillary enlargement, not miosis. The degree of ptosis is usually much more severe in third-nerve palsy than in Horner syndrome; this is because CN III supplies the levator palpebrae, the primary levator of the lid, whereas the sympathetics supply Müller's muscle, which plays an accessory role. The sympathetic pathway does exit the spinal cord at T1, but injury at this location would not cause orbital pain, which is typical of carotid arterial dissection.

18. The answer is a. *(Lee, p 2.)* Computed tomographic scanning measures the density of intracranial as well as extracranial structures. Bone appears much denser than blood, but blood is obvious on the unenhanced (precontrast) CT scan precisely because it is much denser than white matter, gray matter, and CSF. The resolution of the CT scan is generally not sufficient to differentiate the pia mater from the gray matter on which it lies. Other meningeal structures, such as the dura mater, may appear denser than brain, especially if there is some calcification in the membranes.

19. The answer is c. *(Victor, p 1452.)* After injury to the facial nerve, regenerating fibers may be misdirected. This is especially common with Bell's palsy (idiopathic facial weakness). Aberrant regeneration is possible only if the nerve cell bodies survive the injury and produce axons that find their way to neuromuscular junctions. Fibers intended for the periorbital muscles end up at the perioral muscles, and signals for eye closure induce mouth retraction. With a habit spasm or idiopathic tic, similar movements may occur, but the movement disorder would not be linked to facial weakness.

20. The answer is b. *(Victor, pp 888–893.)* This patient gives a good history for subarachnoid hemorrhage. A CT scan will detect blood locally or diffusely in the subarachnoid spaces or within the brain or ventricular system in more than 90% of cases. It is more sensitive than an MRI in most cases and can be obtained more quickly. A cerebral angiogram could diagnose the etiology of a subarachnoid hemorrhage, such as an aneurysm. However, it is an invasive test and should not be done without first attempting to confirm the diagnosis with less risky tests. If you suspect seizures, an electroencephalogram might be useful. As this patient did not have any loss of consciousness, personality changes, hallucinations, or rhythmic movements suggestive of seizures, there is no indication for a psychiatry consult.

21. The answer is b. (*Victor, pp 892–893.*) In suspected subarachnoid hemorrhage, CT will detect blood locally or diffusely in more than 90% of cases. However, if no blood is seen, the physician should proceed to a lumbar puncture. Elevated CSF RBCs, xanthochromia, and increased opening pressure all may be caused by subarachnoid hemorrhage. A cerebral angiogram could diagnose the etiology of a subarachnoid hemorrhage, such as an aneurysm; however, it is an invasive test and should not be done without first attempting to confirm the diagnosis with less risky tests. An MRI is unlikely to give new useful information in this case. Zolmitriptan is a treatment for migraines. This patient's history is not typical for a migraine.

22. The answer is a. (*Victor, p 893.*) This patient probably has a subarachnoid hemorrhage and must be evaluated for an aneurysm. This does not appear to be bacterial meningitis. It is not emergent that ceftriaxone be given in this case. Sumatriptan is a treatment for migraine, and this patient's history and cerebrospinal fluid results do not support a diagnosis of migraine. Repeating the lumbar puncture will not help with the diagnosis or treatment. Intravenous acyclovir would be used to treat herpes encephalitis. Although there are often red blood cells in the spinal fluid of such patients, the overall history makes herpes encephalitis unlikely.

23. The answer is e. (*Victor, p 24.*) Computed tomographic scanning is especially sensitive to intracerebral hemorrhage, but not to aneurysms unless they are more than 5 mm across. Even such relatively large aneurysms may not be revealed by CT scanning unless there is bleeding from the aneurysm or distortion of adjacent structures by the aneurysm. Microscopic aneurysms may be localizable on CT only because of the high signal left near the aneurysm by telltale blood. In most cases of aneurysmal bleeding, angiography is needed to characterize and localize the lesion. The resolution of PET, MRI, SPECT, and CT of intracranial aneurysms is too poor to enable surgical correction of the lesion to proceed without demonstration of the aneurysm on angiography.

24. The answer is a. (*Greenberg, pp 337–338, 597.*) The open black arrow denotes the aqueduct of Sylvius, which connects the third ventricle with the fourth ventricle. This sagittal view of the lower part of the brain provides a high-resolution view of the posterior fossa. What appears to be a connection between the most inferior aspect of the fourth ventricle and the cisterna magna (at the straight black arrow) is an artifact. This is the obex of the fourth ventricle, and there is a complete roof over this ventricle, which communicates with the subarachnoid space through the foramens of Luschka and Magendie.

25. The answer is e. (*Lee, pp 140–148.*) Bone has low signal on this T1-weighted image of the head, the cerebellar tonsil is sitting above the opening of the foramen magnum. The bone marrow in the occipital bone may be seen as high signal (white). With Arnold-Chiari malformations, the tonsil would be expected to sit below the foramen magnum. With Dandy-Walker syndrome or giant cisterna magna, the tonsil would be inapparent or at least sitting much more cephalad.

26. The answer is a. (*Lee, p 107.*) All five of the tumors listed are common in the posterior fossa. The tentorium cerebelli is a fold of meninges. Consequently, it is a relatively common site for the development of meningiomas. A tumor arising on the tentorium may extend either superiorly or inferiorly. Inferior extension of the tumor may damage cranial nerves and make complete extirpation of this benign neoplasm impossible.

27. The answer is b. (*Victor, pp 18–21.*) Calcified masses appear hyperdense without contrast enhancement, whereas highly vascular lesions may appear dense on CT scanning after the patient has received intravenous contrast material. Tumors, granulomas, and other intracranial lesions enhance because of a breakdown in the blood-brain barrier. More cystic lesions may exhibit enhancement limited to the periphery of the cyst.

28. The answer is c. (*Victor, pp 692–693.*) Any type of stroke in the cerebellum would be expected to evolve over the course of hours, rather than days or weeks. With signs and symptoms that evolve slowly, a neoplasm is more likely. Because there was no involvement of the eighth cranial nerve, the most probable neoplasm is a meningioma. This tumor also appears to arise from bone, another indication that it is most likely a meningioma.

29. The answer is c. (*Victor, pp 692–693.*) Complete resection of this large meningioma is probably impractical because of the damage to cranial nerves that would be sustained with any attempt at complete extirpation. If tumor must be left behind, repeated surgery may be necessary. Chemotherapy is not helpful because these tumors are notoriously insensitive. Radiation therapy is controversial because some tumors may become more anaplastic after radiation, but the current evidence supports irradiating residual tumor.

30. The answer is e. (*Victor, pp 692, 1075.*) Meningiomas occur with increased frequency in type 2 neurofibromatosis, a dominantly inherited disorder arising with a deletion on the long arm of chromosome 22. Women with breast cancer and other gynecologic cancers are also at increased risk of developing meningiomas, perhaps because of sex steroid receptors on these tumors that enhance their growth when gynecologic disturbances occur. Estrogen or progesterone antagonists may be useful in the management of these tumors, but tamoxifen, an estrogen inhibitor, paradoxically stimulates the growth of meningioma cells.

31. The answer is c. (*Victor, pp 93–94.*) Dysdiadochokinesia is usually apparent with cerebellar damage. It is most evident when strength and sensation are intact. Alternately tapping one side of the hand and then the other, or tapping the heel and then alternating with the toe of the foot, is the test usually employed to check this aspect of coordination. Multiple sclerosis in adults and cerebellar tumors in children are two of many causes of problems with this part of the neurologic examination. Focal lesions in the nervous system may produce highly asymmetric dysdiadochokinesia. A variety of movement disorders, such as parkinsonism and choreoathetosis, may interfere with rapid alternating movements and give the false impression that the patient has a lesion in systems solely responsible for coordination.

32. The answer is c. (*Victor, pp 27–32.*) The relaxed adult man or woman exhibits α wave activity at a frequency of 8 to 13 Hz over the posterior aspects of the head; α activity disappears with eye opening and with concentration on mathematical activities. This brain wave activity should be equally well developed over both sides of the head. As the subject becomes drowsy, the α activity becomes less obvious.

33. The answer is a. (*Victor, pp 504–514.*) The patient has a tumor in the left frontal-parietal-temporal region. This area is critical for language. This particular patient presented with a Wernicke-type aphasia (impaired naming and comprehension and repetition with fluent speech). Neglect and left hemiparesis would be more likely with right brain lesions. A left homonymous hemianopia would be caused by an occipital lesion on the right side. Alexia without agraphia is a disconnection syndrome associated with lesions involving the left occipital lobe and splenium of the corpus callosum.

34. The answer is i. (*Kasper, p 2386.*) This man has suffered an acute cerebrovascular event. The most important test in the immediate period is a CT scan of the head to establish whether the lesion is hemorrhagic or ischemic. If there is no evidence of hemorrhage on head CT, then the patient is within the 3-h time window permitting therapy with intravenous recombinant tissue plasminogen activator (r-TPA), which has been shown to improve functional outcome after stroke.

35. The answer is c. (*Victor, pp 1354–1358.*) A nerve conduction study should confirm that this woman has a peripheral neuropathy—that is, a disturbance of sensory and motor nerve function in the limbs. Given her social condition, she is at high risk for a nutritional neuropathy. A glove-and-stocking pattern of sensory disturbance is usually seen with lesions that involve peripheral nerves, specifically the nerves extending out into the limbs. The meaning of glove-and-stocking is self-evident: sensation is disturbed over the hands and the feet with extension up the arms and the legs being quite variable. With severe neuropathy of the hands or the feet, ulcerations and pressure sores will develop over the skin that is innervated by the damaged nerves. The most severe sensory deficit affects the most terminal elements of the limbs. Metabolic or nutritional problems are the usual causes of a glove-and-stocking pattern of sensory disturbance. Diabetes mellitus, thiamine deficiency, and neurotoxin damage (e.g., that caused by some insecticides) are the commonest causes of these sensory disturbances. Affected persons usually report the sensation of pins and needles in the hands and feet, but with some neuropathies severe pain may develop along with the loss of sensory acuity.

36. The answer is e. (*Victor, p 335.*) This boy is probably having generalized absence seizures. The EEG will probably show the typical 3-Hz spike-and-wave pattern characteristic of this type of seizure disorder. Even if this patient does not have the typical pattern, the character of his episodes suggests epilepsy (i.e., a tendency to have recurrent seizures), and the EEG should help characterize the type of epilepsy. Because a structural lesion could cause seizures, although not typically generalized absence seizures, an MRI or CT of the head should be performed to establish that no correctable lesion is present.

37. The answer is d. (*Swaiman, pp 982–983.*) Seizures associated with fever at this age are worrisome and must be aggressively investigated. The neck stiffness, fever, and recurrent seizures necessitate a spinal tap to allow examination of the cerebrospinal fluid. The fluid should be checked for the opening pressure, Gram staining, protein and glucose content, cell count, bacterial and fungal cultures, acid-fast bacillus (AFB) staining, and flagellated treponemal antigen (FTA-ABS). Antibiotic treatment should be started immediately if there is any indication of an infection. *Haemophilus influenzae* was commonly responsible for meningitis at this early age prior to the availability of vaccination against it, but infections with a variety of bacteria, including gram-negative bacteria, are also possible causes of the clinical scenario described.

38. The answer is f. (*Victor, pp 1486–1487.*) This patient probably has a myopathy. The elevated ESR and periungual telangiectasias suggest an inflammatory myopathy, and specifically dermatomyositis. Creatine phosphokinase would help to confirm that this is a primary muscle disease. Additional tests that will be of use are electromyography (EMG) and muscle biopsy. Electromyography may show brief, low-voltage action potentials, fibrillation potentials, positive sharp waves, polyphasic units, and some evidence of denervation. Muscle biopsy may show changes characteristic of the particular inflammatory myopathies. In polymyositis, extensive necrosis of muscle fiber segments is seen with macrophage and lymphocyte infiltration. In dermatomyositis, the picture is quite different: there is perifascicular muscle fiber atrophy, and the inflammatory infiltrate occurs in the perimysial connective tissue rather than throughout the muscle fibers themselves. In addition, electron microscopy shows characteristic tubular aggregates. In the rarer inclusion body myositis, the appearance is similar to that of polymyositis except that rimmed vacuoles are also seen.

39. The answer is f. (*Victor, pp 12–18.*) This CSF profile is essentially normal. With idiopathic seizures, the CSF should be normal. Seizure activity does not ordinarily drive up the CSF protein content or significantly change the cellular content of the fluid. Occasionally, there is a mild pleocytosis of up to 80 cells/μL, which peaks 1 day postictally. The acidosis that is observed in this patient is inconsequential and is routinely found during the early postictal period after a generalized tonic-clonic seizure.

40. The answer is d. *(Victor, pp 740–741.)* This man with fever, generalized seizure, lethargy, cough, headache, blurred vision, and progressive stupor probably has acute bacterial meningitis. Given his age of 72 and history of probable upper respiratory infection, a pneumococcal meningitis is highly probable. In bacterial meningitis, the CSF typically exhibits elevated protein content, no or few RBCs, an elevated opening pressure, milky or xanthochromic fluid, and a normal or slightly elevated gamma globulin content. If there are relatively few white cells and the CSF protein is not greatly elevated, the fluid may appear clear and colorless. The WBC count will be elevated, and the WBCs in the CSF will consist of both polymorphonuclear cells and lymphocytes. A very low CSF glucose content supports the diagnosis of bacterial meningitis. Tuberculous meningitis, however, produces an atypical pattern of CSF changes distinct from that caused by other bacterial pathogens and reminiscent of that caused by fungi.

41. The answer is b. *(Victor, p 1382.)* This young man with ascending paralysis with preserved sensation and sphincter control has Guillain-Barré syndrome. His CSF is largely normal except for its markedly high protein. The CSF is xanthochromic (i.e., yellow) because of the high protein content of the fluid. Despite the pattern of weakness, which suggests an ascending myelitis, his CSF reveals a normal cell count. The CSF protein with Guillain-Barré syndrome may exceed 1 g, becoming so viscous that normal CSF flow patterns are disturbed.

42. The answer is g. *(Victor, pp 892–893, 941.)* This man, involved in an automobile accident, probably has subarachnoid blood associated with his head trauma. This is suggested by his neck stiffness, photophobia, and vomiting. That he had transient loss of consciousness and that there was obvious trauma to his head supports the notion that he sustained enough of a blow to his head to produce intracranial bleeding of some sort. Even if the neuroimaging studies do not reveal any contusion, he could still have a substantial accumulation of blood in the subarachnoid space from damage to vessels in the arachnoid itself. A high CSF protein content and xan-thochromia suggest that much of the blood in the CSF has already broken down by the time of the tap. Many RBCs will persist for days with a sub-stantial subarachnoid hemorrhage. The WBC count will be elevated because the subarachnoid blood is irritating and produces a chemical meningitis. The opening pressure may be slightly elevated if there has been much bleeding into the subarachnoid space.

43. The answer is e. (*Victor, pp 793–794.*) This young woman with pro-gressive behavioral disturbances, hallucinations, seizures, and obtundation probably has a herpes simplex type 1 encephalitis. The CSF with herpes simplex encephalitis often has some RBCs in addition to the primarily mononuclear increase in WBCs. The CSF protein is elevated, but the glu-cose content is relatively normal with this viral infection. As the CSF pro-tein increases, the percentage that is gamma globulin generally increases. This is not an indication that the problem is an infection, but this increase in total protein and gamma globulin component does occur with infec-tions. The opening pressure may be markedly elevated, but the fluid may remain clear or be only slightly cloudy if the white blood cell count does not increase substantially.

44. The answer is c. (*Victor, pp 968–969.*) This young man has signs and symptoms of multiple sclerosis that are largely referable to the spinal cord. Gait ataxia is an especially common presenting complaint. Impotence is troublesome and common. The CSF fluid picture is distinctive in its eleva-tion of the gamma globulin content. Oligoclonal banding studies of the fluid would most likely be positive.

45. The answer is a. (*Victor, pp 667–668.*) This woman with headaches, papilledema, and slightly blurred vision probably has pseudotumor cere-bri. This idiopathic increase in intracranial pressure usually occurs in obese young women, during pregnancy, or with hypervitaminosis. The extraordi-narily high CSF opening pressure associated with pseudotumor cerebri does not produce herniation of the brain, and performing a spinal tap does not place the patient at increased risk for transforaminal herniation. The CSF glucose content, protein content, cell count, and gamma globulin studies in persons with pseudotumor cerebri should all be unremarkable.

Cerebrovascular Disease

Questions

DIRECTIONS: Each item below contains a question followed by suggested responses. Select the **one best** response to each question.

46. A 67-year-old woman with a history of type 2 diabetes mellitus and atrial fibrillation presents to the emergency room with left body weakness and slurred speech. The onset was sudden while she was brushing her teeth 1 h ago, and she was brought immediately to the emergency room. She denies word-finding difficulties, dysesthesia, and headache. She is taking warfarin. Physical exam findings include blood pressure of 205/90 and irregularly irregular heartbeat. There is left side neglect with slurred speech. There is a corticospinal pattern of weakness of the left body, with the face and upper extremity being worse than the lower extremity. Routine chemistries and cell counts are normal. Her INR is 1.8. Which of the following is the most appropriate first step in management?

a. Administer tissue plasminogen activator
b. Call a vascular surgery consult for possible endarterectomy
c. Order a brain CT
d. Order a cerebral angiogram
e. Start heparin

47. A patient is diagnosed with an acute stroke. A right middle cerebral artery occlusion is demonstrated by magnetic resonance angiogram shown below. Which of the following is the most common cause of stroke?

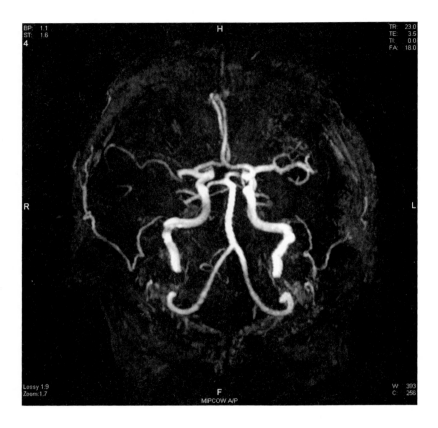

a. Atherosclerosis
b. Fibromuscular dysplasia
c. Mitral valve prolapse
d. Arterial dissection
e. Meningovascular inflammation

48. A pure motor stroke is most likely with damage to which of the following?

a. Internal capsule
b. Cerebellum
c. Putamen
d. Caudate
e. Amygdala

49. A pure sensory stroke is most likely with damage to which of the following?

a. Internal capsule
b. Thalamus
c. Hippocampus
d. Globus pallidus
e. Pons

50. A 61-year-old man with a history of hypertension has been in excellent health until he presents with vertigo and unsteadiness lasting for 2 days. He then develops nausea, vomiting, dysphagia, hoarseness, ataxia, left facial pain, and right-sided sensory loss. There is no weakness. On examination, he is alert, with a normal mental status. He vomits with head movement. There is skew deviation of the eyes, left ptosis, clumsiness of the left arm, and titubation. He has loss of pin and temperature sensation on the right arm and leg and decreased joint position sensation in the left foot. He is unable to walk. Magnetic resonance imaging (MRI) in this patient might be expected to show which of the following?

a. Basilar artery tip aneurysm
b. Right lateral medullary infarction
c. Left lateral medullary infarction
d. Left medial medullary infarction
e. Right medial medullary infarction

51. A 50-year-old man had a brainstem stroke following a vertebral artery dissection secondary to an acute sports-related injury. This patient might be expected to develop dysphagia secondary to involvement of which of the following structures?

a. Nucleus solitarius
b. Nucleus and descending tract of CN V
c. Nucleus ambiguus
d. Lateral spinothalamic tract
e. Inferior cerebellar peduncle

52. Occlusion of which of the following arteries typically produces Wallenberg (lateral medullary) syndrome?

a. Basilar artery
b. Vertebral artery
c. Superior cerebellar artery
d. Anterior inferior cerebellar artery (AICA)
e. Anterior spinal artery

53. A 75-year-old man with a history of recent memory impairment is admitted with headache, confusion, and a left homonymous hemianopsia. He has recently had two episodes of brief unresponsiveness. There is no history of hypertension. Computed tomography (CT) scan shows a right occipital lobe hemorrhage with some subarachnoid extension of the blood. An MRI scan with gradient echo (susceptibility) sequences reveals foci of hemosiderin in the right temporal and left frontal cortex. Which of the following is the most likely cause of this patient's symptoms and signs?

a. Gliomatosis cerebri
b. Multi-infarct dementia
c. Mycotic aneurysm
d. Amyloid angiopathy
e. Undiagnosed hypertension

54. A 22-year-old male abuser of intravenous heroin has been having severe headaches during sexual intercourse. Within a few minutes of one headache, he develops right-sided weakness and becomes stuporous. His neurologic examination reveals neck stiffness as well as right arm and face weakness. An unenhanced emergency CT scan reveals a lesion of 3 to 4 cm in the cortex of the left parietal lobe. The addition of contrast enhancement reveals two other smaller lesions in the right frontal lobe but does not alter the appearance of the lesion in the left parietal lobe. Which of the following diagnostic studies is most likely to establish the basis for this patient's neurologic deficits?

a. HIV antibody testing
b. Cerebrospinal fluid (CSF) examination
c. Electroencephalography
d. Nerve conduction studies
e. Cardiac catheterization

55. A 52-year-old right-handed woman who has abused intravenous drugs for many years has an HIV antigen test that is positive. CD4+ (helper) T lymphocyte count is normal. A brain CT scan reveals several hemorrhagic lesions. Nerve conduction studies reveal generalized slowing in the legs, and EEG exhibits focal slowing over the left parietal lobe. Cardiac catheterization suggests aortic valve disease, and the patient's CSF is xanthochromic (yellow). Which of the following is the probable site of injury in the CNS?

a. An arterial wall
b. The ventricular endothelium
c. The pia arachnoid
d. The dura mater
e. The perivenular space

56. A 35-year-old man presented to the emergency room with the acute onset of right body weakness. A diffusion-weighted MRI was positive and is in part shown below. Further imaging sequences indicated a small left frontal intraparenchymal hemorrhage. Within 1 day of admission, the patient's right-sided weakness began to abate, and within 1 week it almost completely resolved. On the sixth day of hospitalization, the patient abruptly lost consciousness and exhibited clonic movements starting in his right side and generalizing to his left side. The movements stopped within 3 min, but he had residual right-sided weakness for 24 h. A head CT scan was unchanged from admission. The most appropriate treatment to institute involves which of the following?

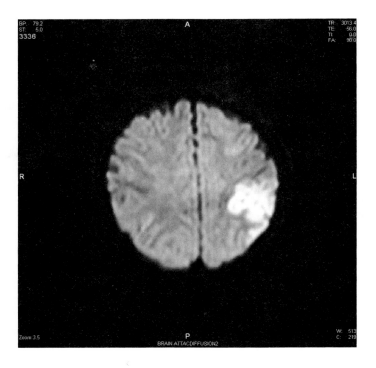

a. Heparin
b. Recombinant tissue plasminogen activator (r-TPA)
c. Lamotrigine
d. Phenytoin
e. Warfarin

57. Focal weakness lasting for 24 h following a motor seizure is most likely attributable to which of the following?

a. Intracerebral hemorrhage
b. Subarachnoid hemorrhage
c. Encephalitis
d. Todd's paralysis
e. Hyponatremia

58. A 16-year-old girl with complex partial seizures and mild mental retardation has an area of deep red discoloration (port-wine nevus) extending over her forehead and left upper eyelid. A CT scan of her brain would be likely to reveal which of the following?

a. A hemangioblastoma
b. A Charcot-Bouchard aneurysm
c. An arteriovenous malformation
d. A leptomeningeal angioma
e. A fusiform aneurysm

59. A 72-year-old woman has the abrupt onset of right face and hand weakness, disturbed speech production, and a right homonymous hemianopsia. This is most likely attributable to occlusion of which of the following arteries?

a. Left middle cerebral artery
b. Left anterior cerebral artery
c. Left vertebrobasilar artery
d. Right anterior choroidal artery
e. Left posterior inferior cerebellar artery (PICA)

60. A 39-year-old woman has diplopia several times a day for 6 weeks. She consults a physician when the double vision becomes unremitting, and also mentions a dull pain behind her right eye. When a red glass is placed over her right eye and she is asked to look at a flashlight off to her left, she reports seeing a white light and a red light. The red light appears to her to be more to the left than the white light. Her right pupil is more dilated than her left pupil and responds less briskly to a bright light directed at it than does the left pupil. Before any further investigations can be performed, the woman develops the worst headache of her life and becomes stuporous. Her physician discovers that she has marked neck stiffness and photophobia. The physician performs a transfemoral angiogram. This radiologic study is expected to reveal that the woman has which of the following?

a. An arteriovenous malformation
b. An occipital astrocytoma
c. A sphenoidal meningioma
d. A pituitary adenoma
e. A saccular aneurysm

61. A 43 year-old man presents with a left CN III deficit and headache. Which of the following is the most likely site of the lesion responsible for this presentation?

a. Anterior communicating artery
b. Posterior communicating artery
c. Anterior cerebral artery
d. Middle cerebral artery
e. Posterior cerebral artery

62. Three days after a subarachnoid hemorrhage, a patient begins to develop neck stiffness and photophobia. This is followed by left-sided weakness and hyperreflexia. Her left plantar response is upgoing. Her physician presumes that these deficits are a delayed effect of the subarachnoid blood. Which of the following is the most appropriate treatment?

a. Heparin
b. Warfarin
c. Nimodipine
d. Phenytoin
e. Carbamazepine

63. A 73-year-old man with a history of hypertension has a 10-min episode of left-sided weakness and slurred speech. On further questioning, he relates three brief episodes in the past month of sudden impairment of vision affecting the right eye. His examination now is normal. Which of the following is the most appropriate next diagnostic test?

a. Creatine phosphokinase (CPK)
b. Holter monitor
c. Visual evoked responses
d. Carotid artery Doppler ultrasound
e. Conventional cerebral angiography

64. Episodes of visual loss known as amaurosis fugax are most likely related to which of the following?

a. Retinal vein thrombosis
b. Central retinal artery ischemia
c. Posterior cerebral artery ischemia
d. Middle cerebral artery ischemia
e. Posterior ciliary artery ischemia

65. A thorough evaluation reveals that a 69-year-old patient has a symptomatic 90% stenosis of the right internal carotid artery at the bifurcation. Which of the following management options is most likely to prevent a future stroke?

a. Warfarin
b. Carotid artery angioplasty
c. Carotid endarterectomy
d. Extracranial-intracranial bypass
e. Aspirin

DIRECTIONS: Each group of questions below consists of lettered options followed by a set of numbered items. For each numbered item, select the **one** lettered option with which it is **most** closely associated. Each lettered option may be used once, more than once, or not at all.

Questions 66–74

For each clinical scenario, pick the language disturbance that best explains the clinical picture.

a. Broca's aphasia
b. Wernicke's aphasia
c. Transcortical sensory aphasia
d. Transcortical motor aphasia
e. Anomic aphasia
f. Global aphasia
g. Conduction aphasia
h. Mixed transcortical aphasia

66. A 62-year-old man with a history of myocardial infarction awakens with a dense right-sided hemiplegia. His eyes are tonically deviated to the left, and he does not respond to threat on the right side of his visual field. He appears to be alert and responds to pain on the left side of his body. His speech is unintelligible and nonfluent, and he follows no instructions. Efforts to get him to repeat simple phrases consistently fail.

67. A 45-year-old woman with chronic atrial fibrillation discontinues warfarin treatment and abruptly develops problems with language comprehension. She is able to produce some intelligible phrases and produces sound quite fluently; however, she is unable to follow simple instructions or to repeat simple phrases. On attempting to write, she becomes very frustrated and agitated. Emergency MRI reveals a lesion of the left temporal lobe that extends into the superior temporal gyrus.

68. A 71-year-old man develops headache and slight difficulty speaking while having sexual intercourse. He has a long-standing history of hypertension, but has been on medication for more than 7 years. He makes frequent errors in finding words and follows complex commands somewhat inconsistently. The most obvious defect in his language function is his inability to repeat the simplest of phrases without making repeated errors.

An emergency CT scan reveals an intracerebral hemorrhage in the left parietal lobe that appears to communicate with the lateral ventricle.

69. A 24-year-old woman abruptly loses all speech during the third trimester of an otherwise uncomplicated pregnancy. She has a history of severe migraines during which she occasionally develops a transient right hemiplegia. Her comprehension is good, and she is frustrated by her inability to speak or write. She is unable to repeat simple phrases, but she does begin to produce simple words within 5 days of the acute disturbance of language.

70. A 78-year-old man has a cardiac arrest while being treated in an emergency room for chest pain. Resuscitation is initiated immediately, but profound hypotension is observed for at least 20 min. A cardiac rhythm is restored, but the patient remains unconscious for the next 3 days. When he is awake, alert, and extubated, his speech is limited to repetition of words and sounds produced by those around him. He has no apparent comprehension of language and produces few sounds spontaneously. Whenever the patient is spoken to, he fairly accurately repeats what was said to him.

71. A 62-year-old man has had a left hemisphere stroke. He has impaired naming and repetition. His speech is nonfluent. Comprehension is preserved.

72. An 82-year-old man has had a slow, stepwise cognitive deterioration. A brain MRI is consistent with the diagnosis of dementia due to multiple cerebral infarcts. Naming is impaired. Comprehension, repetition, and fluency are relatively maintained.

73. A 53-year-old woman sustains a small left frontal embolic stroke during cardiac catheterization. She has poor naming ability and is nonfluent. Comprehension and repetition are relatively preserved.

74. A 28-year-old woman is hit in the left neck while playing lacrosse. Approximately 2 hours later she begins having language difficulties. Her speech is fluent and nonsensical. She cannot understand commands, but repeats well.

Cerebrovascular Disease

Answers

46. The answer is c. (*Victor, p 824.*) This is a good history for cardioembolic stroke—sudden onset, cortical symptoms, atrial fibrillation, and subtherapeutic INR. The immediate goal should be to rule out an intracranial hemorrhage and confirm the diagnosis. Tissue plasminogen activator is the treatment for acute stroke in specific circumstances. However, it is not yet certain that this is a stroke. It may be an intracranial hemorrhage, which would be a contraindication for tissue plasminogen activator. Additionally, an elevated INR in a patient on warfarin is a contraindication for tissue plasminogen activator. Carotid endarterectomy is indicated for some cases when a transient ischemic attack or stroke is believed to be caused by carotid artery narrowing. It is not yet known what caused this patient's event, and this procedure would rarely be done emergently. A cerebral angiogram would be indicated if there was a strong suspicion of an aneurysm or vascular malformation. There is no reason to believe one of these is causing the patient's symptoms. Heparin may be indicated if there is not an intracranial hemorrhage. This must first be established by CT or MRI.

47. The answer is a. (*Victor, p 825.*) Atherosclerosis may produce cerebral infarction by a variety of mechanisms, including emboli to the brain and local occlusion of atheromatous vessels. Platelet emboli may form on ulcerated atheromatous plaques in major vessel walls and ascend to the brain. The atherosclerotic plaque involves subintimal proliferation of smooth muscle, fatty deposits in the intima, inflammatory cells, and excessive elaboration of the connective tissue matrix in the vessel wall. Thrombi may form on the surface of the plaque and occlude the vessel, even if the plaque is not large enough to produce substantial narrowing of the vessel. Fibromuscular dysplasia is a relatively uncommon cause of cranial vessel occlusion that develops with segmental overgrowth of fibrous and muscular tissue in the media. Meningovascular inflammation is a rare process that occurs in some infectious or inflammatory disorders, such as syphilis, tuberculous meningitis, or sarcoid.

48. The answer is a. (*Victor, p 831.*) Pure motor deficits are especially likely in hypertensive persons with small infarctions, called *lacunae*. The pure motor stroke is the most common type of lacunar stroke. The affected person usually has hemiplegia unassociated with cognitive, sensory, or visual deficits. The posterior limb of the internal capsule is the usual site of injury. The lacunae are assumed to develop because of an occlusive lesion in an arteriole that supplies the injured structure.

49. The answer is b. (*Victor, p 839.*) Pure sensory strokes are most likely in the same persons who are susceptible to pure motor strokes and other lacunae. With hypertensive injury to the posteroventral nucleus of the lateral thalamus, the affected person will report contralateral numbness and tingling. During recovery from this type of stroke, paradoxical pain may develop in the area of sensory impairment. This paradoxical pain associated with decreased pain sensitivity is referred to as the *thalamic pain syndrome*.

50. The answer is c. (*Victor, pp 844–846.*) Wallenberg, or lateral medullary, syndrome is due to infarction involving some or all of the structures located in the lateral medulla, including the nucleus and descending tract of the fifth nerve, the nucleus ambiguus, lateral spinothalamic tracts, inferior cerebellar peduncle, descending sympathetic fibers, vagus, and glossopharyngeal nerves. The patient with Wallenberg syndrome has ipsilateral ataxia and ipsilateral Horner syndrome. The trigeminal tract damage may produce ipsilateral loss of facial pain and temperature perception and ipsilateral impairment of the corneal reflex. The lateral spinothalamic damage produces pain and temperature disturbances contralateral to the injury in the limbs and trunk. Dysphagia and dysphonia often develop with damage to the ninth and tenth nerves.

51. The answer is c. (*Victor, pp 844–845.*) The nucleus ambiguus, located in the ventrolateral medulla, contains the motor neurons that contribute to the ninth (glossopharyngeal) and tenth (vagus) cranial nerves. The motor neurons of the nucleus ambiguus innervate the striated muscles of the larynx and pharynx as well as provide the preganglionic parasympathetic supply to thoracic organs, including the esophagus, heart, and lungs. Injury to this nucleus and its pathways causes hoarseness and dysphagia.

52. The answer is b. (*Victor, pp 842–846.*) Most cases of lateral medullary infarction are due to occlusion of the vertebral artery. Several small branches of the distal vertebral artery supply the lateral medulla. In some cases, occlusion of the posterior inferior cerebellar artery (PICA) causes this syndrome. The PICA is the last large branch of the vertebral artery, and, when it is occluded, there may also be infarction of the inferior cerebellum accompanying that of the medulla.

53. The answer is d. (*Lee, pp 190, 581–582.*) Cerebral amyloid angiopathy (CAA), or congophilic angiopathy, is the most common cause of lobar hemorrhage in elderly patients without hypertension. The deposition of β-amyloid protein (the same as that found in Alzheimer's disease) in brain blood vessels leads to disruption of the vessel walls, which predisposes them to hemorrhage. Patients are usually over age 70 and may present with multiple cortical hemorrhages, with or without a history of dementia. At times, additional hemorrhages may be seen only on special imaging techniques, such as gradient echo MRI, which magnifies the effects of hemosiderin in regions of prior hemorrhage.

54. The answer is b. (*Victor, pp 902–903.*) This young man almost certainly has numerous problems associated with his intravenous drug abuse, but the cause of his current problems is most likely bleeding from a mycotic aneurysm. Aneurysms are especially likely to bleed during exertion, such as that associated with sexual intercourse or defecation. The fact that the lesion appeared largely the same on unenhanced and enhanced CT scans suggests that it is a hematoma. HIV antibody testing might reveal evidence of exposure to HIV, but, aside from establishing that the patient was at increased risk of opportunistic infections, that test would provide little insight into the cause of the acute neurologic syndrome. The CSF would be expected to be xanthochromic (yellow), with many (>20/μL) red blood cells (RBCs), or grossly bloody, thereby providing evidence of a recent subarachnoid hemorrhage. Electroencephalography would undoubtedly reveal an asymmetric pattern associated with the left hemispheric lesion, but this too would provide little insight into the cause of the problem. Nerve conduction studies would not clarify the basis for a lesion of the central nervous system, because they examine only structures of the peripheral nervous system. Cardiac catheterization might reveal valvular abnormalities, but these need not be associated with disease of the central nervous system.

55. The answer is a. (*Victor, pp 902–903.*) The most likely explanation for this patient's deficits is bleeding from a mycotic aneurysm. This type of aneurysm is usually relatively small and might not be evident on CT scanning or even on arteriography. An arteriogram would miss the lesion if it had destroyed itself when it bled or if the aneurysmal sac was completely thrombosed. The name *mycotic* is misleading. It suggests a fungal etiology, but it actually refers to the appearance of these aneurysms, which tend to be multiple. These aneurysms occur with either gram-positive or gram-negative infections, but the responsible organisms usually have relatively low virulence. Mycotic aneurysms form over the cerebral convexities with subacute bacterial endocarditis. The aneurysm develops from an infected embolus originating on the diseased heart valves and lodging in the arterial wall. Bleeding from these small aneurysms is largely directed into the subarachnoid space. More virulent organisms that produce valvular heart disease are more likely to produce a meningitis or multifocal brain abscess with seeding of infected emboli to the brain. With acquired immune deficiency syndrome (AIDS), a fungus could be the causative agent, but patients with endocarditis more typically have streptococcal or staphylococcal infections. Even if mycotic aneurysms form with endocarditis, they need not inevitably become symptomatic.

56. The answer is d. (*Victor, pp 356–360.*) Anticoagulation with warfarin or heparin and thrombolysis with r-TPA or urokinase are contraindicated in anyone with an intracranial hemorrhage. Focal seizures that secondarily generalize after an intracerebral or subarachnoid hemorrhage occur frequently and are appropriately treated with an antiepileptic drug, such as phenytoin (Dilantin). Lamotrigine is an anticonvulsant, but would be a very poor choice in this case because this patient needs a drug that will be immediately therapeutic. Lamotrigine must be slowly titrated over many weeks when first started because of the risk of severe rash.

57. The answer is d. (*Victor, pp 345–346.*) Weakness after seizure activity is evidence of a postictal paralysis, or Todd's paralysis. Postictal weakness does not suggest bleeding or new areas of cerebrocortical damage, but imaging with CT scan is appropriate to exclude these possibilities. Postictal paralysis may last for many hours, or even days. The precise cause is unknown, but it appears to be due to some kind of neuronal exhaustion occurring after frequent repetitive discharges. It may reflect depletion of glucose in the neurons in the epileptic focus.

58. The answer is d. (*Greenberg, p 601. Victor, pp 1077–1078.*) This patient has encephalofacial angiomatosis (Sturge-Weber syndrome), a congenital disturbance that produces facial cutaneous angiomas with a distinctive and easily recognized appearance, along with intracranial abnormalities such as leptomeningeal angiomas. Persons with the syndrome may be mentally retarded and often exhibit hemiparesis or hemiatrophy on the side of the body opposite the port-wine nevus. Both men and women may be affected, and seizures may develop in affected persons. The nevus associated with Sturge-Weber syndrome usually extends over the sensory distribution of the first division of the trigeminal nerve. The lesion usually stays to one side of the face. Affected persons will usually also have an angioma of the choroid of the eye. Intracranial angioma is unlikely if the nevus does not involve the upper face. Deficits develop as the person matures and may be a consequence of focal ischemia in the cerebral cortex that underlies the leptomeningeal angioma. Hemangioblastomas are vascular tumors seen in association with polycystic disease of the kidney and telangiectasias of the retina (von Hippel-Lindau syndrome). Charcot-Bouchard aneurysms are very small and may be microscopic. They develop in patients with chronic hypertension and most commonly appear in perforating arteries of the brain. The lenticulostriate arteries are most commonly affected. Hemorrhage from these aneurysms is likely, and the putamen is the most common site for hematoma formation. Hemorrhage may extend into the ventricles and lead to subarachnoid blood. Other locations commonly affected include the caudate nucleus, thalamus, pons, and cerebellum. The dentate nucleus of the cerebellum is especially susceptible to the formation of Charcot-Bouchard aneurysms. Fusiform aneurysms are diffusely widened arteries with evaginations along the walls, but without stalks as occur with the typical berry-shaped structures of the saccular aneurysm. This type of aneurysm may be a late consequence of arteriosclerotic damage to the artery wall.

59. The answer is a. (*Victor, pp 834–835.*) The left middle cerebral artery supplies the cortex around the sylvian fissure, as well as some of the frontal lobe structures involved in speech. The optic radiation loops through the temporal lobe on its way to the occipital cortex and is usually damaged with occlusion of the middle cerebral artery. The speech disorder likely with an injury of the left frontal lobe is a Broca's aphasia. Comprehension would be expected to be largely intact, but if the patient has damage to enough of the temporal lobe cortex, a Wernicke's aphasia might develop. Choroidal artery occlusions might produce focal weakness, but speech problems would be less likely. Occlusion of the PICA can produce a variety of brainstem and cerebellar signs, but this combination of deficits would be unlikely with a lesion outside the cerebral cortex.

60. The answer is e. (*Victor, pp 890–892.*) The clinical picture suggests that a saccular aneurysm has become symptomatic by compressing structures about the base of the brain and subsequently leaking. Aneurysms enlarge with age and usually do not bleed until they are several millimeters across. Persons with intracerebral or subarachnoid hemorrhages before the age of 40 are more likely to have their hemorrhages because of arteriovenous malformations than because of aneurysms. Aneurysms occur with equal frequency in men and women below the age of 40; however, in their forties and fifties, women are more susceptible to symptomatic aneurysms. This is especially true of aneurysms that develop on the internal carotid on that segment of the artery that lies within the cavernous sinus. An angiogram is useful in establishing the site and character of the aneurysm. A CT scan would be more likely to reveal subarachnoid, intraventricular, or intraparenchymal blood, but it would reveal the structure of an aneurysm only if it were several (>5) millimeters across. An MRI will reveal relatively large aneurysms if the system is calibrated and programmed to look at blood vessels. This patient had a transfemoral angiogram, a technique that involves the introduction of a catheter into the femoral artery; the catheter is threaded retrograde in the aorta and up into the carotid or other arteries of interest.

61. The answer is b. (*Victor, pp 888–892.*) An aneurysm on the posterior communicating artery is especially likely to compress the oculomotor (third) nerve. Because the pupilloconstrictor fibers lie superficially on this nerve, problems with pupillary activity are routinely early phenomena. An ischemic injury to the third cranial nerve, such as that seen with diabetes mellitus, will usually spare these superficial fibers, presumably because they have a vascular supply that is fairly distinct from that of the rest of the third nerve. The pupillary response to both direct and consensual stimulation will be impaired with compression of these parasympathetic nerve fibers. This means that the pupil in the right eye will not constrict in response to light shining into either the right or the left eye. The normal pupil on the left will constrict with light shining into either the left or the right eye because the sensory input from the right eye is unimpaired. As the aneurysm enlarges, it impinges upon the third-nerve fibers that supply the medial rectus muscle, weakness of which will be responsible for double vision. Lesions of the superior cerebellar artery and posterior cerebral artery can also compress the third nerve, which exits between them. It is therefore important that a complete angiogram, evaluating all four vessels, be performed in the evaluation for subarachnoid hemorrhage and third-nerve palsy.

62. The answer is c. *(Victor, pp 894–895.)* Vasospasm is a relatively common complication of subarachnoid blood and may result in stroke. Nimodipine is used because it decreases the probability of stroke, but it does not prevent it completely. Anticoagulation with heparin or warfarin worsens the patient's prospects because it increases the risk of additional bleeding. Antiepileptic drugs, such as phenytoin and carbamazepine, may reduce the risk of seizure associated with subarachnoid blood and are sometimes given prophylactically. This patient does not have evidence of seizures, however.

63. The answer is d. *(Victor, pp 859–860.)* This patient is experiencing the classical symptoms of extracranial internal carotid artery disease, which include episodes of ipsilateral transient monocular blindness (amaurosis fugax) and contralateral transient ischemic attacks consisting of motor weakness. Patients with symptomatic extracranial carotid artery disease have a high likelihood of going on to develop strokes (approximately 26% over 2 years on medical therapy). The appropriate test to confirm the suspicion of carotid stenosis is a Doppler ultrasound of the carotid arteries. This test utilizes the fact that sound waves will bounce back from particles moving in the bloodstream—primarily red blood cells—at a different frequency depending on the velocity and direction of the blood flow. A great deal of important information about the structure of the blood vessel can be obtained in this way. Although angiography can also provide this information, it is invasive, carries a risk of causing a stroke, and is more expensive.

64. The answer is b. *(Victor, pp 254–256.)* The presumed mechanism of transient monocular blindness in carotid artery disease is embolism to the central retinal artery or one of its branches. Although classic teaching has emphasized the role that cholesterol emboli play in causing this blindness, it has been noted that cholesterol emboli (Hollenhorst plaques) may be seen on funduscopic examination even of asymptomatic individuals. Retinal vein thrombosis may produce a rapidly progressive loss of vision, with hemorrhages in the retina, but would not be associated with the transient attacks of amaurosis fugax. Although both posterior and middle cerebral artery ischemia can cause visual loss, they would not be expected to cause the monocular blindness of amaurosis fugax. Posterior ciliary artery ischemia can cause ischemic optic neuropathy, but this is usually acute, painless, and not associated with preceding transient monocular blindness or TIAs.

65. The answer is c. *(Victor, pp 867–868.)* Based on the results of the North American Symptomatic Carotid Endarterectomy Trial (NASCET), it is known that carotid endarterectomy can reduce the risk of stroke in patients with symptomatic stenosis by 70% or more. The risk of ipsilateral stroke was reduced from 26% in the medically treated group to 9% in the surgically treated group. Carotid endarterectomy should be offered to all eligible patients with symptomatic disease of the internal carotid artery. There is currently no randomized, controlled trial data to support the use of warfarin, carotid angioplasty, or stenting in the management of these patients, although studies of angioplasty are under way. Extracranial-intracranial bypass has been tried unsuccessfully, although it may still play a role for certain patients with inaccessible lesions or hypoperfusion in the setting of complete occlusions. Aspirin would be appropriate after endarterectomy.

66. The answer is f. *(Victor, pp 504–515.)* Given the patient's history of cardiovascular disease, one must suspect that this man has sustained a stroke of the left cerebral hemisphere. Either the left internal carotid artery or the left middle cerebral artery is probably occluded. The area of infarction would be expected to include the frontal, temporal, and parietal lobe cortices. The tonic gaze deviation indicates damage to the frontal lobe center on the left, which directs the eyes contralaterally. The right visual field loss occurs with damage to the optic radiation in the left hemisphere.

67. The answer is b. *(Victor, pp 504–515.)* Presumably, an embolus from this woman's heart traveled to a branch of the middle cerebral artery that supplied her dominant hemisphere. The left hemisphere is usually the speech-dominant hemisphere. Wernicke's aphasia is the most common of the so-called fluent aphasias: the affected person produces a string of sounds that may sound like a real language, but the sounds are generally meaningless. The patient seems to be unaware that his or her speech is incomprehensible. Comprehension and repetition are impaired. Typically, efforts at speaking produce only a meaningless string of phonemes that retain the rhythm and intonation of normal speech.

68. The answer is g. *(Victor, pp 504–515.)* According to one classic model of language organization formulated by the neurobehaviorist Norman Geschwind, the expressive language centers in the frontal lobe and the receptive centers in the temporal lobe communicate in large part along the arcuate fasciculus, which extends through the temporal and parietal lobes. This man appears to have suffered an acute hemorrhage associated with chronic hypertension. The blood extended into the lateral ventricle, which was the probable cause of the headache. Patients with the rare syndrome of conduction aphasia have problems with repetition that are more obvious than their problems with comprehension. Their speech usually does not sound very fluent.

69. The answer is a. *(Victor, pp 504–515.)* Cerebrovascular occlusions are unusual at the age of 24, but this woman had two risk factors for stroke: her migraine headaches and her pregnancy. The stroke probably involved the frontal lobe cortex about the third frontal convolution on the dominant side. Speech becomes telegraphic (i.e., consisting of short phrases with omission of small connecting words such as articles and conjunctions) with a Broca's aphasia, but permanent loss of all ability to produce meaningful language is unlikely if the area of infarction is less than a few centimeters across. The most persistent difficulty usually exhibited by patients with this type of stroke is a permanent loss of syntax.

70. The answer is h. (*Victor, pp 504–515.*) With protracted hypotension, this patient suffered a watershed infarction. The cortex at the limits of the supply of the principal cerebral arteries was inadequately perfused, and the resulting infarction isolated the speech areas in the frontal and temporal lobes from the cortex in other parts of the cerebrum. Language usually does not recover substantially after this type of infarction.

71. The answer is a. (*Victor, pp 504–515.*) Broca's is the classic anterior (nonfluent) aphasia and is characterized as described in the question. It is most often assocoated with a lesion of the left inferior frontal gyrus.

72. The answer is e. (*Victor, pp 504–515.*) Anomic aphasia consists of an isolated word-finding deficit. It is the least localizable of the major aphasias. It is common in patients with diffuse brain dysfunction.

73. The answer is d. (*Victor, pp 504–515.*) Transcortical motor aphasia is similar to Broca's aphasia with the exception of preserved repetition. Anatomically, the lesion generally occupies left frontal white matter and spares the overlying cortex.

74. The answer is c. (*Victor, pp 504–515.*) Transcortical sensory aphasia is similar to Wernicke's aphasia with the exception of preserved repetition. Anatomically, the lesion generally occupies the white matter underlying the cortex of Wernicke's area. In most cases, the prognosis for improvement is better than for that of Wernicke's aphasia.

Epilepsy and Seizures

Questions

DIRECTIONS: Each item below contains a question followed by suggested responses. Select the **one best** response to each question.

75. A 9-year-old boy is brought to your clinic by his parents because he has begun to have episodes of eye fluttering lasting several seconds. Sometimes he loses track of his thoughts in the middle of a sentence. There was one fall off a bicycle that may have been related to one of these events. There are no other associated symptoms, and the episodes may occur up to 20 or more times per day. The boy's development and health have been normal up until this point. He did have two head injuries as a young child: the first when he fell off a tricycle onto the ground, and the second when he fell off of a playset onto his head. Both episodes resulted in a brief loss of consciousness and he did not think clearly for part of the day afterward, but had no medical intervention. Which of the following tests is most likely to confirm this patient's diagnosis?

a. Brain CT scan
b. Brain MRI
c. Electroencephalogram
d. Lumbar puncture
e. Nerve conduction study

76. A 19-year-old right-handed man who carries the diagnosis of epilepsy is seen in the urgent care clinic. He had been healthy until about age 12, when he began to have episodes of eye fluttering lasting several seconds. Sometimes he would lose track of his thoughts in the middle of a sentence. There was one fall off of a bicycle that may have been related to one of these events. He has been treated with valproic acid. At one point he was off all medications, but the seizures returned. He is now at the end of his first semester of college and came in today because he had a witnessed generalized tonic-clonic seizure this morning. He had had only about 2 hours of sleep the night before because he was studying for a final exam. Which of the following is the most appropriate thing to tell this patient?

a. "I know that you faked this seizure to avoid taking a test."
b. "Lack of sleep may have contributed to triggering this seizure."
c. "You can expect to have tonic-clonic seizures on a regular basis from now on."
d. "Your seizures are getting worse and there is nothing we can do about it."
e. "You should take the next semester off to recover and get extensive testing."

77. A 56-year-old man with epilepsy is brought into the emergency room. He has been having continuous generalized tonic-clonic seizures for the past 30 min. He is treated with 2 mg of intravenous lorazepam. Most physicians recommend using a high dose of intravenous benzodiazepine as part of the management of status epilepticus because it has which of the following qualities?

a. Ability to suppress seizure activity for more than 24 h after one injection
b. Lack of respiratory depressant action
c. Rapid onset of action after intravenous administration
d. Lack of hypotensive effects
e. Lack of dependence on hepatic function for its metabolism and clearance

78. A 34-year-old woman is having her medications tapered in the epilepsy monitoring unit. She has a convulsive seizure that does not stop after 5 min, even after she receives a lorazepam injection. A second intravenous drug is given. Infusing which of the following antiepileptic drugs at more than 50 mg/min in an adult may evoke a cardiac arrhythmia?

a. Carbamazepine
b. Diazepam
c. Phenobarbital
d. Clonazepam
e. Phenytoin

79. A 44-year-old man presents with left arm shaking. Two days ago, the patient noticed left arm paresthesias along the lateral aspect of his left arm and left fourth and fifth fingers while he was reading. He thinks he may have been leaning on his left arm at the time; the symptoms resolved after 30 seconds. This morning, he noted the same feelings, lasting a few seconds, but then his fourth and fifth fingers started shaking rhythmically, and the shaking then spread to all of his fingers, his hand, and then his arm up to his elbow. This episode lasted a total of 30 seconds. He denies any strange smells or tastes, visual changes, or weakness. Afterward, his fingers felt locked in position for a few seconds. Then he felt as if he did not have control of his hand and had difficulty donning his socks. He and his wife decided to drive to emergency room, and in the car he had trouble putting his seat belt latch into its socket. Examination and routine labs are normal. Which of the following is the most appropriate next action?

a. Discharge the patient to follow up in clinic in 2 weeks
b. Obtain a brain MRI
c. Obtain an electroencephalogram
d. Obtain an orthopedic consult
e. Order electromyography and nerve conduction studies

80. A 31-year-old right-handed woman has a history of alcohol abuse requiring detox. Currently, she says she is drinking about nine beers 3 days per week. She drank five glasses of wine and three beers 5 days ago. Last night, she had 10 beers. This morning, she awoke feeling well. She was speaking with her fiancé, went to the bathroom, and got back into bed. She had no headache, fever, chills, nausea, vomiting, or pain. Suddenly her body became stiff with arms flexed for a few seconds, followed by rhythmic jerking of both arms. Her legs were shaking, but less so. Her eyes were open, and she was foaming at the mouth. After 1 min, this stopped, and she initially did not recognize her fiancé or his sister. She slowly returned to a normal level of consciousness over a 10-minute period. She remembers events just prior to the episode, and she remembers being in the car on the way to the hospital. Her only medication is a multivitamin. She denies illicit drugs. Her examination is entirely normal. Routine labs and a brain MRI are normal. Which of the following is the most likely underlying cause of her condition?

a. Autoimmune
b. Genetic
c. Infectious
d. Neoplastic
e. Toxic/metabolic

81. A 4-year-old boy has the onset of episodes of loss of body tone, with associated falls, as well as generalized tonic-clonic seizures. His cognitive function has been deteriorating. EEG shows 1.5- to 2-Hz spike-and-wave discharges. Which of the following is the most likely diagnosis?

a. Landau-Kleffner syndrome
b. Lennox-Gastaut syndrome
c. Juvenile myoclonic epilepsy
d. Mitochondrial encephalomyopathy
e. Febrile seizures

82. A 27-year-old man begins to experience infrequent episodes of nausea, warmth rising through his body, and an unusual odor like rotting fish. His girlfriend notices that afterward he may develop twitching of the left side of his face and an inability to speak for several minutes. Afterward the man appears dazed and cannot remember what has occurred. He has otherwise been well. Magnetic resonance imaging (MRI) of his brain is most likely to show a lesion in which of the following areas?

a. Left occipital lobe
b. Right frontal lobe
c. Cribriform plate
d. Uncus
e. Left parietal lobe

83. An 18-year-old girl riding on the back of her boyfriend's motorcycle without a helmet is brought in with a left frontal skull fracture and cortical contusion. GCS is 10. She is admitted to the intensive care unit. She has had no seizures. Which of the following is true regarding anticonvulsant therapy in this case?

a. It is contraindicated due to risk of rash
b. It is best achieved using phenobarbital
c. It is likely to cause increased cerebral edema
d. It is indicated to reduce the incidence of late posttraumatic epilepsy
e. It is indicated to reduce the incidence of early posttraumatic seizures

84. A patient with intractable complex partial seizures due to cortical dysplasia undergoes left temporal lobectomy. He is most likely to develop which of the following problems after surgery?

a. Right superior quadrantanopsia
b. Right inferior quadrantanopsia
c. Right homonymous hemianopsia
d. Right hand weakness
e. Aphasia

85. A 29-year-old man with a history of febrile seizures as a child has developed medication refractory complex partial seizures within the past 2 years. An MRI reveals the abnormality indicated by the arrow. Which of the following is true regarding this condition?

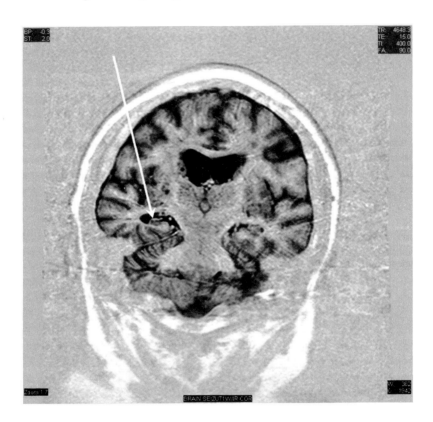

a. This patient may benefit from a neurosurgical procedure
b. The patient will probably die within 2 years
c. The seizures will most likely stop with further medication titration
d. A head CT should be performed
e. A cerebral angiogram may confirm the diagnosis

DIRECTIONS: Each group of questions below consists of lettered options followed by a set of numbered items. For each numbered item, select the **one** lettered option with which it is **most** closely associated. Each lettered option may be used once, more than once, or not at all.

Questions 86–91

For each clinical scenario, choose the seizure type that best explains the patient's complaints.

a. Generalized tonic-clonic
b. Generalized absence
c. Complex partial
d. Epilepsia partialis continua
e. Simple partial sensory
f. Jacksonian march
g. Psychomotor status
h. Tonic-clonic status epilepticus
i. Pseudoseizures
j. Myoclonic

86. A 37-year-old man develops involuntary twitching movements in his left thumb. Within 30 s, he notices that the twitching has spread to his entire left hand and that involuntary movements have developed in his left forearm and the left side of his face. He cannot recall what happened subsequently, but his wife reports that he fell down and the entire left side of his body appeared to be twitching. He appeared to be unresponsive for about 3 min and confused for another 15 min. During the episode, he bit his tongue and wet his pants.

87. A 17-year-old boy reports involuntary jerking movements in his arms when he awakens. This has occurred during the day after a nap as well as in the morning after a full night's sleep. Over the next few months, he developed similar jerks during the day, even when he had been awake for several hours. He did not lose consciousness with these muscle jerks, but did occasionally fall. On one occasion, jerks in his legs caused a fall that resulted in a fractured wrist.

88. A 21-year-old man reports several episodes over the previous 4 years during which he lost consciousness. He had no warning of the impending episodes, and with each episode he injured himself. Observers told him that he abruptly developed a blank stare and stopped talking. His body became stiff and he arched his back. After several seconds of this type of posturing, his arms and legs started shaking violently. During one of these episodes, he dislocated his right shoulder. He routinely bit his tongue and urinated in his pants during the episodes.

89. A 25-year-old woman was fired from her job after she misplaced papers vital for the company. She had had recurrent episodes for several years during which she performed nonsensical activities such as burying her plates in the backyard, hiding her underwear, and discarding her checkbook. She did not recall what she had done after performing these peculiar activities. She had been referred for psychotherapy, but the episodes became even more frequent after she was started on thioridazine (Mellaril). Her husband observed one episode and noted that she was unresponsive for about 5 min and confused for at least 1 h. She did not fall down or remain immobile during the episodes. As the episodes became more frequent, she noticed that she would develop an unpleasant taste in her mouth, reminiscent of motor oil, just before an episode.

90. A 21-year-old cocaine-abusing man develops seizures that persist for more than 30 min before emergency medical attention is available. When examined nearly 1 h later, he is still exhibiting tonic-clonic movements and has never recovered consciousness.

91. A 16-year-old boy with a history of acute viral myocarditis requires placement of a left ventricular assist device. He has a complicated postoperative course, with fever, bacteremia, and renal failure. On postoperative day 10, he develops continuous rhythmic jerking of the left corner of the mouth, associated with jerking of the left thumb. This persists for 24 h. He is alert, able to follow commands, and has no gaze deviation. Computed tomography shows a small hemorrhagic infarction of the right posterior frontal region.

Questions 92–95

For each clinical scenario, choose the medication(s) that is most appropriate in the management of the patient's problem.

a. Lorazepam
b. Magnesium sulfate
c. Clonazepam
d. Felbamate
e. Phenobarbital
f. Carbamazepine
g. Divalproex sodium
h. Primidone
i. Lamotrigine
j. Adrenocorticotropic hormone (ACTH)

92. A 19-year-old woman describes recurrent memory problems. Her fiancé reports that she seems to be inattentive for minutes at a time several times a week. She never injures herself during these episodes, but she cannot recall what happened, and, on one occasion, she became lost while walking home. An ambulatory EEG demonstrates evolving spike activity originating in the left temporal lobe during one of the episodes. The EEG pattern does not generalize. Computed tomography and MRI scanning of the brain reveal no structural abnormalities. Conversations with the woman's parents reveal that she had febrile seizures when she was 3 years old, which abated with antipyretic treatment alone.

93. A 7-month-old boy develops generalized limb extension and neck flexion spasms that occur more than 20 times daily and are associated with altered consciousness. EEG reveals diffuse, high-voltage, polyspike-and-slow-wave discharges between spasms and suppression of these bursts during the spasms. A sibling died with a brainstem glioma, and the father has several large areas of hypopigmented skin in the shape of ash leaves. The infant had obvious psychomotor retardation even before the appearance of the spasms.

94. A 5-year-old girl has frequent staring spells and does not respond when her mother calls her name during these episodes. She never falls down or bites her tongue, but she does have occasional lip smacking during episodes. EEG reveals a 3/s (Hz) spike-and-wave pattern that occurs for less than 10 s at a time but several times an hour. The child has normal motor and cognitive development.

95. A 35-year-old pregnant woman at term is admitted to the hospital for delivery. She has headaches and visual blurring. Her blood pressure is 180/100. On examination, she is edematous. Reflexes are increased. Protein is found in the urine. She then develops a generalized tonic-clonic convulsion.

Epilepsy and Seizures

Answers

75. The answer is c. *(Victor, p 335.)* This is a common presentation for primary generalized epilepsy of childhood. An electroencephalogram showing the classic 3-Hz spike-and-wave pattern would confirm this diagnosis. Brain MRI and CT are useful for evaluating brain anatomy. Anatomic problems can cause seizures, but these tests will not provide any information about brain electrical activity. Lumbar puncture is useful for measuring cerebrospinal fluid pressure and looking for central nervous system inflammation or infection. Central nervous system inflammation or infection may cause seizures. Nerve conduction study is useful to evaluate peripheral nerve injuries such as nerve entrapment.

76. The answer is b. *(Bradley, p 2025.)* Lack of sleep is a common seizure trigger. There is no reason to believe that the patient faked the seizure. It is impossible to predict his future seizure course based on this one event; having one seizure does not necessarily mean that his seizures are getting worse, and even if they are, many treatments are available. There is no reason for the patient to take a prolonged leave of absence from school because of one seizure. This may even have detrimental psychological consequences.

77. The answer is c. *(Bradley, pp 1968–1969.)* Until recently, the most popular benzodiazepine for use in status epilepticus was diazepam (Valium), which has a rapid onset of action but is cleared relatively quickly. Because of this property, patients needed additional medications, such as phenytoin, to protect them from recurrent seizure activity as early as 20 min after diazepam injection. A longer-acting benzodiazepine, lorazepam (Ativan), has the advantage of acting rapidly like diazepam but being cleared more slowly from the brain.

78. The answer is e. *(Bradley, p 1968.)* Rapid infusion of phenytoin may produce a cardiac arrhythmia or hypotension. Phenytoin should not be administered at rates greater than 50 mg/min in adults or 1 mg/(kg·min) in children to reduce the chances of this reaction occurring. Thus, it usually requires approximately 20 min to administer a 1000- to 1500-mg standard loading dose of phenytoin in an emergent setting such as status epilepticus. Fosphenytoin, a water-soluble prodrug of phenytoin, has the advantage of causing fewer infusion site reactions. It can be given at doses of up to 150 mg/min in an adult, with risks of cardiac dysrhythmia similar to those of phenytoin. Another advantage of fosphenytoin is that it can be administered intramuscularly when intravenous access is problematic. Carbamazepine is not administered intravenously at all. Rapid infusion of phenobarbital may produce hypotension or respiratory arrest, but is much less likely to depress cardiac activity. Diazepam and clonazepam are safer than phenobarbital, but rapid infusion of excessively high doses may depress blood pressure and other autonomic functions.

79. The answer is b. *(Bradley, pp 1976–1978.)* This history is typical of a simple partial seizure. A focal brain lesion must be ruled out. It would be wrong to discharge the patient to follow up in clinic in 2 weeks without at least a CT scan and preferably an MRI. Although he probably had a seizure, obtaining an electroencephalogram at this point will not be as helpful as an MRI. This is unlikely to be a peripheral nerve problem, and therefore an orthopedic consult or electromyography and nerve conduction studies are not indicated.

80. The answer is e. *(Victor, pp 1239–1242.)* This is a typical example of alcohol withdrawal seizure. The greatest risk for alcohol withdrawal seizures occurs within the first day after drinking cessation, in contrast to delirium tremens, which usually occurs within 2 to 4 days of drinking cessation. There is no evidence of an autoimmune process in this patient. Rasmussen encephalitis is an example of a seizure disorder thought to be of autoimmune etiology. There are many examples of genetically transmitted epilepsies, which usually present during childhood. Infections such as meningitis, brain abscess, or encephalitis can cause seizures. Signs of these include meningeal signs, fever, and MRI findings. If this patient had a brain tumor, you might expect a history of headache due to increased intracranial pressure. Additionally, the exam and MRI would likely be abnormal.

81. The answer is b. *(Bradley, p 1966.)* Lennox-Gastaut syndrome is characterized by mental dysfunction, multiple seizure types and 1- to 2-Hz generalized spike-wave discharges on EEG. It is often difficult to control the seizures that develop in children with this syndrome. Many affected children have a history of infantile spasms (West syndrome). Infants and children with infantile spasms exhibit paroxysmal flexions of the body, waist, or neck and usually have a profoundly disorganized EEG pattern called *hypsarrhythmia*.

82. The answer is d. *(Victor, p 338.)* Many patients with complex partial seizures have a preseizure phenomenon (the aura) that alerts them to an impending seizure. This patient's aura includes an olfactory hallucination, which is usually associated with lesions of the mesial temporal lobe, particularly the uncus or parahippocampal gyrus. Diseases that can affect that region include tumors, trauma, and mesial temporal sclerosis.

83. The answer is e. *(Victor, p 944.)* There is evidence that prophylactic phenytoin reduces the incidence of seizures after head injury. Because early posttraumatic seizures may lead to increased morbidity and prolonged hospital stays, it is reasonable in some situations to treat patients prophylactically. There is no evidence that prophylactic treatment reduces the long-term risk of developing posttraumatic epilepsy.

84. The answer is a. *(Patten, p 25.)* The most common complication of temporal lobectomy is a visual field defect due to interruption of fibers from the optic tracts passing over the temporal horn of the lateral ventricles. Superior quadrantanopsia is more common than hemianopsia. Some deficits may improve if the injury does not completely damage the nerves. Language deficits, particularly dysnomia, occur less frequently. Hemiparesis is uncommon (<2%), because the surgery is performed at a distance from the motor fibers of the corticospinal tract. Other neurological problems that can occur include diplopia due to extraocular nerve deficits, and facial paresis.

85. The answer is a. *(Bradley pp 1972–1973.)* The history and MRI are typical for mesial temporal sclerosis (MTS). The arrow in the MRI is specifically pointing at the sclerotic right hippocampus. This is the most common cause of intractable complex partial seizures in adults. The prognosis for improved seizure control with additional medications is poor; however surgical resection of the right anterior temporal lobe may produce seizure freedom in up to 80% of cases. If this patient had a high-grade malignant brain tumor, he would probably die within 2 years. A cerebral angiogram may confirm the diagnosis of a vascular malformation.

86. The answer is f. (*Victor, pp 337–338.*) With a Jacksonian march, or sequential seizure, the patient develops focal seizure activity that is primarily motor and spreads. This type of seizure often secondarily generalizes, at which point the patient loses consciousness and may have a generalized tonic-clonic seizure. The hand is a common site for the start of a Jacksonian march. The face may be involved early because the thumb and the mouth are situated near each other on the motor strip of the cerebral cortex.

87. The answer is j. (*Victor, p 109.*) Myoclonic seizures may be generalized or partial. They are most commonly seen in the epilepsy syndrome called *benign juvenile myoclonic epilepsy* (BJME). Unlike sleep myoclonus, the episodes occur when the affected person wakes up rather than when he or she is falling asleep. Myoclonic jerks may be triggered by light flashes or loud sounds. Benign juvenile myoclonic epilepsy accounts for 4% of all cases of epilepsy. More than half of those with BJME have generalized tonic-clonic seizures as well as myoclonic seizures.

88. The answer is a. (*Victor, pp 333–334.*) With generalized tonic-clonic seizures, the EEG develops abnormalities all over the cortex simultaneously. The patient may recall a strange sensation before the attack, but it is equally likely that no premonitory sign or aura will occur. Partial seizures may secondarily generalize to this type of seizure. If the patient has frequent generalized tonic-clonic seizures, he or she will be at high risk for a variety of injuries, such as dislocated shoulders, broken bones, and head trauma. Patients with this type of seizure always lose consciousness during the attack and may be confused for minutes or hours after the ictus, the most obvious segment of the seizure.

89. The answer is c. (*Victor, pp 339–342.*) Complex partial seizures may be mistaken for a psychiatric problem, especially if the partial seizures do not generalize and produce tonic-clonic seizures. This patient has a typical aura involving an unpleasant smell or taste. These were once called *uncinate fits,* because they were ascribed to abnormal activity in the uncus of the temporal lobe. Complex partial seizures may arise from a focus of abnormal electrical activity in the temporal lobe, but they do not invariably arise from a temporal lobe focus.

90. The answer is h. *(Bradley, pp 1967–1970.)* Status epilepticus is defined as a seizure that lasts continuously for 30 min or a series of seizures over a 30-min period without the patient's regaining full consciousness between them. Status constitutes a medical emergency, because the longer the seizures last, the worse the morbidity and mortality. Complications of status include respiratory failure, aspiration, acidosis, hypotension, rhabdomyolysis, renal failure, and cognitive impairment.

91. The answer is d. *(Victor, pp 343–344.)* Epilepsia partialis continua refers to a condition of persistent focal motor seizure activity—in essence, a focal motor status epilepticus. The distal hand and foot muscles are most frequently affected. Active or passive movement of the limb may exacerbate the seizure activity. The seizures may persist for hours or for months. The response to therapy is often poor.

92. The answer is f. *(Victor, pp 356–360.)* This young woman is having complex partial seizures without secondary generalization. She has episodic altered consciousness associated with a temporal lobe seizure focus and antedated by febrile seizures. Carbamazepine is the best choice because of its relatively good adverse effect profile in persons in this age group.

Phenytoin is another reasonable option, but carries with it the adverse effects of hirsutism and gingival hypertrophy, often considered undesirable in a young woman. Because she is of childbearing age, the patient has the additional problem of a slightly increased risk of birth defects in her offspring. However, the risk to the fetus from seizure activity is probably greater than that from exposure to an antiepileptic drug.

93. The answer is j. *(Victor, p 342.)* This child has West syndrome, a generalized seizure disorder of infants characterized by recurrent spasms, the EEG pattern of hypsarrhythmia, and retardation. Several different diseases cause West syndrome. The family history in this case suggests tuberous sclerosis as the underlying problem. Adrenocorticotropic hormone is the best of the given choices.

94. The answer is g. *(Victor, p 360.)* This girl has generalized absence attacks. This may be a manifestation of a more complex epilepsy syndrome or may occur as an isolated finding. Generalized absence attacks have no aura and no postictal period. The affected child has no warning that an attack is about to occur and is usually unaware that one has occurred unless it is more than a few seconds long. In fact, generalized absence seizures are most often only a few seconds long. Ethosuximide is the drug of choice, but it may cause gastrointestinal distress. Divalproex sodium is effective in many of the children who cannot tolerate ethosuximide or who are not well controlled on that antiepileptic. If the absence seizures are associated with generalized tonic-clonic seizures, divalproex sodium is a better choice.

95. The answer is b. *(Bradley, pp 2544–2545.)* Recent studies have established that magnesium sulfate ($MgSO_4$) is the optimal treatment both to prevent seizures in women with hypertension at the time of admission for delivery (preeclampsia) and to treat seizures in established eclampsia. The dose is 4 to 5 g intravenously, followed by a 1-g/h intravenous infusion. Magnesium sulfate was shown to result in a reduction in recurrent seizures and in maternal morbidity and mortality compared with both diazepam and phenytoin. In addition, the fetus should be delivered as quickly as possible, using C-section if necessary.

Headache and Facial Pain

Questions

DIRECTIONS: Each item below contains a question followed by suggested responses. Select the **one best** response to each question.

96. A 22-year-old woman reports a scotoma progressing across her left visual field over the course of 30 min, followed by left hemicranial throbbing pain, nausea, and photophobia. Her brother and mother have similar headaches. Which of the following is present in classic migraine but not in common migraine?

a. Photophobia
b. Familial pattern
c. Visual aura
d. Hemicranial pain
e. Nausea

97. A 16-year-old woman has been having attacks of weakness, blurry vision, and loss of consciousness. Following consultation with a neurologist, the diagnosis of basilar migraine is made. Basilar migraine differs from classic migraine in which of the following ways?

a. Sex of the persons most often affected
b. Resistance of the visual system to involvement
c. Severity of symptoms
d. Duration of the aura
e. Sequence of neurologic deficits and headache

98. A 43-year-old woman describes lancinating pains radiating into the right side of her jaw. This discomfort has been present for more than 3 years and has started occurring more than once a week. The pain is paroxysmal and routinely triggered by cold stimuli, such as ice cream and cold drinks. She has sought relief with multiple dental procedures and has already had two teeth extracted. Multiple neuroimaging studies reveal no structural lesions in her head. Assuming there are no contraindications to the treatment, a reasonable next step would be to prescribe which of the following?

a. Clonazepam (Klonopin), 1 mg orally three times daily
b. Diazepam (Valium), 5 mg orally two times daily
c. Divalproex sodium (Depakote), 250 mg orally three times daily
d. Indomethacin (Indocin), 10 mg orally three times daily
e. Carbamazepine (Tegretol), 100 mg orally three times daily

99. A 23-year-old woman has had 1 week of worsening facial pain. She describes it as an intense shooting pain that comes and goes. It is present only on her right face. Which of the following is most likely to be this patient's underlying problem?

a. Multiple sclerosis
b. Tolosa-Hunt syndrome
c. Migraine
d. Anterior communicating artery aneurysm
e. Falx meningioma

100. A 39-year-old left-handed woman is being treated with carbamazepine for lancinating pain in her left face. The pain is paroxysmal, usually occurring without apparent reason, but seems sometimes to be brought on by a cold breeze. Both trigeminal neuralgia and atypical facial pain involve pain that may be which of the following?

a. Lancinating
b. Paroxysmal
c. Associated with anesthetic patches
d. Abolished with resection of the gasserian ganglion
e. Unilateral

101. A 26-year-old graduate student presents to the emergency room with a severe left-sided throbbing headache associated with nausea, vomiting, and photophobia. She has tried taking ibuprofen without relief. On further questioning, she relates that she has been having similar headaches three to four times per month for the past year. Her mother had a similar problem. Her exam is normal. Appropriate therapy for this patient's present headache might include which of the following drugs?

a. Ergotamine tartrate
b. Nitroglycerine
c. Verapamil
d. Amitriptyline hydrochloride
e. Phenobarbital

102. Appropriate long-term management of a patient with 14 migraine headaches per month might include a prescription for daily use of which of the following medications?

a. Metoclopramide hydrochloride
b. Sumatriptan
c. Oral contraceptives
d. Amitriptyline hydrochloride
e. Ergotamine tartrate

103. A 32-year-old woman is being evaluated for headaches. They started about 6 months ago and occur a few times per week, lasting until she falls asleep. The pain is constant and focused at the front and back of the head. The pain is unrelated to position and tends to be worse later in the day. There is mild photophobia. Which of the following findings is most likely?

a. Slightly reduced neck range of motion and paracervical tenderness
b. Papilledema
c. Abnormal brain MRI
d. Abnormal brain CT
e. Abnormal EEG

DIRECTIONS: Each group of questions below consists of lettered options followed by a set of numbered items. For each numbered item, select the **one** lettered option with which it is **most** closely associated. Each lettered option may be used once, more than once, or not at all.

Questions 104–108

For each clinical scenario, pick the diagnosis that best explains the clinical picture.

a. Classic migraine
b. Cluster headache
c. Common migraine
d. Trigeminal neuralgia
e. Sinusitis
f. Temporal arteritis
g. Vertebrobasilar migraine
h. Hemiplegic migraine
i. Atypical facial pain
j. Postherpetic neuralgia

104. A 22-year-old dance instructor routinely develops headaches on the weekend. The headaches are almost always limited to the right side of her head and centered about the right temple. She knows that a headache is coming because of changes in her vision that precede the headache by 20 to 30 min. She sees scintillating lights just to the left of her center of vision. This visual aberration then expands and interferes with her vision. The blind spot that it creates appears to have a scintillating margin. As the blind spot clears, the headache starts. It rarely lasts more than 1 h, but is usually associated by nausea and vomiting.

105. A 29-year-old woman comes to the emergency room with facial pain of new onset. She has stabbing pains on the left side of her face just below her eye. These last less than 1 s at a time, but are so severe that she winces involuntarily with each pain. The pain seems to be triggered by drinking cold fluids. The only other problems she has noticed are clumsiness in her right hand and blurred vision in her right eye. Both of these have been present for more than 2 years and have not interfered with her normal activities.

106. A 35-year-old man has severe throbbing pain waking him from sleep at night and persisting into the day. This pain is usually centered about his left eye and appears on a nearly daily basis for several weeks or months each year. It occurs most prominently at night within a few hours of falling asleep and is associated with a striking personality change in which the man becomes combative and agitated. He never vomits or develops focal weakness.

107. A 76-year-old man develops a dull left-sided head pain with some radiation of the discomfort to the right side of the head. He has no nausea or vomiting with the pain, but has lost 10 lb over the previous 2 months. His erythrocyte sedimentation rate is 102 mm/h, and he is mildly anemic. An extensive investigation for malignancy reveals no signs of lymphoma, carcinoma, or leukemia.

108. An 81-year-old man with chronic lymphocytic leukemia develops pain and burning over the right side of his face. Within a few days, a vesiculopapular rash in the distribution of the first division of the trigeminal nerve appears. The vesicles become encrusted, and the burning associated with the rash abates. Within 1 month the rash has largely resolved, but the man is left with a dull ache over the area of the rash that is periodically punctuated by shooting pains. Imipramine 100 mg nightly helps reduce the intensity of the chronic pain.

Questions 109–111

For each clinical scenario, select the most likely diagnosis.

a. Carotid artery dissection
b. Pseudotumor cerebri
c. Glioblastoma multiforme
d. Thunderclap headache
e. Analgesic rebound headache
f. Paroxysmal hemicrania
g. Raeder syndrome
h. Intracranial hypotension
i. Posttraumatic headache
j. Aseptic meningitis

109. An obese 37-year-old woman has had a daily headache, worse in the morning, for 1 year. She has episodes of transient visual obscurations affecting each eye, and also hears a pulsatile tinnitus. Examination is notable for bilateral papilledema. There are no other abnormalities.

110. A 42-year-old man presents with a sudden and severe headache associated with nausea. The headache reaches maximal intensity within 5 seconds. He has no prior history of headache. Examination is unremarkable. Computed tomography and spinal fluid examination show no evidence of blood. He later admits that he had been engaged in sexual activity when the headache occurred.

111. A 29-year-old man relates that he has had recent headaches only when standing up. The headaches resolve quickly when he lies down, and are accompanied by mild nausea. His examination is normal.

Headache and Facial Pain

Answers

96. The answer is c. *(Victor, pp 180–181.)* Classic migraine, but not common migraine, is preceded by an aura of neurologic dysfunction. The aura is most often visual in nature, consisting of bright flashing lights, scintillating scotomas, or field cuts. Both kinds of migraine are most often characterized by a hemicranial throbbing headache associated with nausea, vomiting, photophobia, and phonophobia (aversion to sound). Familial patterns are not unusual with either classic or common migraine, although with classic migraine the probability that another family member will have a similar problem approaches 80%.

97. The answer is c. *(Victor, pp 183–184.)* As with classic migraine, with basilar migraine women are more susceptible than men, disturbances of vision are common, the aura usually resolves within 10 to 30 min, and the headache invariably follows, rather than precedes, the neurologic deficits; however, the character and severity of neurologic deficits associated with basilar migraine are distinct. The visual change may evolve to complete blindness. Irritability may develop into frank psychosis. Rather than a mild hemiparesis, the patient may have a transient quadriplegia. Stupor, syncope, and even coma may appear and persist for hours.

98. The answer is e. *(Patten, p 375.)* This woman probably has trigeminal neuralgia (tic douloureux). The treatment options for this facial pain disorder include carbamazepine (Tegretol). Although carbamazepine is a potent antiepileptic medication, other antiepileptic medications, such as phenobarbital and divalproex sodium (Depakote), are usually ineffective in blunting the pain. Phenytoin (Dilantin) is another antiepileptic useful in the management of trigeminal neuralgia, and recently gabapentin (Neurontin) has had some success as well. Analgesics and anti-inflammatory drugs, such as indomethacin (Indocin), are notably ineffective in managing this disorder.

99. The answer is a. (*Victor, p 971.*) Multiple sclerosis is often associated with trigeminal neuralgia, which is then termed *symptomatic trigeminal neuralgia* because it occurs as a symptom of another illness. Other causes of symptomatic trigeminal neuralgia include basilar artery aneurysms, acoustic schwannomas, and posterior fossa meningiomas, all of which may cause injury to the fifth cranial nerve by compression. The Tolosa-Hunt syndrome is a presumably inflammatory disorder that produces ophthalmoplegia associated with headache and loss of sensation over the forehead. Pupillary function is usually spared, and the site of pathology is believed to be in the superior orbital fissure or the cavernous sinus. It is usually not associated with trigeminal neuralgia.

100. The answer is e. (*Victor, pp 196, 200–201.*) Unlike patients with trigeminal neuralgia, who describe paroxysmal, lancinating pains, patients with atypical facial pain usually feel a constant, deep pain. Although atypical facial pain is often bilateral, it may be unilateral and fairly limited in its distribution. The cheek, nose, or zygomatic regions are often affected by this idiopathic pain syndrome. The pain is often sensitive to antidepressant medication, a characteristic that has led some to suggest that the syndrome is invariably caused by depression. Progressive loss of sensation in the distribution of the fifth cranial nerve should prompt a careful search for an underlying malignancy invading the nerve either intracranially or in the face.

101. The answer is a. (*Victor, pp 187–189.*) This patient has common migraine. Of the agents listed, only ergotamine tartrate is generally considered of use to abort a headache. Verapamil and amitriptyline hydrochloride may be used as prophylactic (preventative) therapy. Phenobarbital is an anticonvulsant and is not typically used to treat migraine. Nitroglycerine can actually precipitate headaches in susceptible individuals. Nausea is a frequent accompaniment of migraine. Metoclopramide hydrochloride (Reglan) may be effective in relieving the nausea, but it also reduces gastric stasis, which can retard absorption of oral medications. Certain antiemetics, such as prochlorperazine, may relieve nausea and also provide relief from the headache itself. Additional agents that might be of benefit in abortive therapy include ibuprofen, aspirin, acetaminophen, isometheptene (Midrin), or a triptan. The triptans are a group of medications that act as agonists at serotonergic receptors (specifically, the 5HT-1 receptors), and they have been found to be very effective at stopping migraine headaches.

102. The answer is d. (*Victor, pp 187–189.*) Several medications are effective as prophylactic agents in the treatment of migraine. These include amitriptyline hydrochloride, propranolol, verapamil, and valproate. Most experts recommend initiating prophylactic therapy only when headaches occur at least one to two times per month. Metoclopramide hydrochloride, sumatriptan, and ergotamine tartrate are appropriately used to treat an acute attack of migraine and should not be prescribed on a daily basis. Daily use of these medications can establish a rebound syndrome that results in a chronic daily headache. Oral contraceptives may be associated with either an increase or decrease in the frequency of migraines, but are not generally used as a treatment for migraine. Some experts recommend not prescribing OCPs for patients with migraine for fear of increasing the risk of a stroke, although OCPs are probably safe to use in most patients with common migraine.

103. The answer is a. (*Bradley, pp 2096–2098.*) The history is typical for a tension-type headache. These headaches are often associated with neck muscle spasm leading to reduced neck range of motion and paracervical tenderness. Papilledema and neuroimaging abnormalities would be associated with headaches due to an intracranial mass. The EEG is generally normal in patients with headaches, unless there is underlying damaged brain.

104. The answer is a. (*Victor, pp 182–183.*) Classic migraine is usually familial, involves a unilateral, throbbing head pain, and diminishes in frequency with age. The blind spot, or scotoma, that may develop as part of the aura of a classic migraine attack will involve the same visual field in both eyes. This defect usually changes over the course of minutes. It typically enlarges and may intrude on the central vision. The margin of the blind spot is often scintillating or dazzling. If this margin has a pattern like the battlement of a castle, it is called a *fortification spectrum,* or teichopsia. Homonymous hemianoptic defects of the sort that develop during the aura of a classic migraine indicate an irritative lesion that is affecting one part of the occipital cortex in one hemisphere of the brain. The changes in the scotoma over the course of minutes indicate that the irritative phenomenon sets off a cascade of events in the visual cortex that temporarily disturbs vision in a progressively larger area. Other focal neurologic phenomena may precede classic migraine; the most common are tingling of the face or hand, mild confusion, transient hemiparesis, and ataxia. Fatigue, irritability, and easy distractibility often develop before a migraine. Affected persons usually also have hypersensitivity to light and noise during an attack.

105. The answer is d. (*Victor, pp 196–198.*) Trigeminal neuralgia may develop in the context of multiple sclerosis—an association suggested by this woman's other neurologic problems. The development of trigeminal neuralgia (tic douloureux) indicates that demyelination has probably extended to the brainstem and may be involving trigeminal nerve connections. A more detailed history would probably reveal that the patient has had pain in the eye that now has disturbed vision. This is expected with the optic neuritis, which is typically associated with multiple sclerosis. Other symptoms commonly reported at this age by patients with previously undiagnosed multiple sclerosis include bed wetting (enuresis), changes in speech (dysarthria), and gait instability (ataxia).

106. The answer is b. (*Victor, pp 189–191.*) The term *cluster headache* refers to the tendency of these headaches to cluster in time. They may be distinctly seasonal, but the triggering event is unknown. The pain of cluster headache is usually described as originating in the eye and spreading over the temporal area as the headache evolves. In contrast to migraine, men are more often affected than women, and extreme irritability may accompany the headache. The pain usually abates in less than 1 h. Affected persons routinely have autonomic phenomena associated with the headache that include unilateral nasal congestion, tearing from one eye, conjunctival injection, and pupillary constriction. The autonomic phenomena are on the same side of the face as the pain. These phenomena are similar to those elicited by the local action of histamine and gave rise to the now largely abandoned term *Horton's histamine headaches.*

107. The answer is f. (*Victor, pp 193–194.*) Both men and women are at risk for temporal arteritis, and the greatest risk to both is loss of vision in association with the headache. The erythrocyte sedimentation rate is usually dramatically elevated, and the abolition of symptoms with corticosteroid therapy is equally dramatic. Temporal arteritis is largely nonexistent in persons under 50 years of age and rare in those under 60. Many patients exhibit persistent fevers and progressive weight loss. The temporal arteries are likely to be pulseless or at least thickened. Biopsy of the artery often reveals a giant cell arteritis.

108. The answer is j. *(Victor, pp 198–199.)* The rash preceding the facial pain was probably caused by herpes zoster, a virus that erupts in the severely ill elderly and in immunosuppressed persons. The virus is manifested earlier in life as chickenpox and remains dormant for decades in most people. Tricyclic drugs, such as imipramine hydrochloride, are often more useful than analgesics in suppressing the pain associated with this postviral syndrome.

109. The answer is b. *(Victor, p 194.)* Pseudotumor cerebri, or idiopathic intracranial hypertension, is a condition of unknown cause that results in increased intracranial pressure, predominantly affecting obese women in their childbearing years. Symptoms include headaches, transient visual obscurations, progressive visual loss, pulsatile tinnitus, diplopia, and shoulder and arm pain. Neurological examination shows papilledema or optic atrophy if the syndrome has been long-standing, and occasionally sixth-nerve palsies may be present. Neuroimaging must be performed to exclude mass lesion or venous sinus obstruction, which can also lead to a similar syndrome of intracranial hypertension. Spinal fluid examination should be normal except for an elevated opening pressure. Additional causes of intracranial hypertension include systemic lupus erythematosus, renal disease, hypoparathyroidism, radical neck dissection, vitamin A intoxication, and steroid withdrawal. Treatment options include lumbar puncture, ventriculoperitoneal shunting, and optic nerve sheath fenestration.

110. The answer is d. *(Bradley, p 2063.)* Thunderclap headache refers to the syndrome of the sudden onset of a very severe headache with no apparent structural cause. When a patient presents with "the worst headache of my life," the initial concern should always be for a subarachnoid hemorrhage, particularly in the presence of meningismus, focal deficits, or a change in the level of consciousness. Computed tomography scanning is indicated to exclude hemorrhage, but because CT may be negative in up to 5 to 10% of cases of subarachnoid hemorrhage, lumbar puncture is necessary if CT is negative to exclude small amounts of blood. Some reports have suggested that even in the absence of blood on a lumbar puncture, an underlying aneurysm may still be the cause of acute, severe headache, because sudden changes in the wall of the aneurysm may provoke severe pain. These reports would suggest that angiography should be performed in all such patients to exclude aneurysm. It remains unknown, however, whether these cases represent coincidental occurrence of thunderclap headache and an incidental, asymptomatic aneurysm. Several series have shown that many patients with thunderclap headache tend to go on to develop more typical migraine, raising the possibility that the thunderclap headache is simply the initial presentation of their migraine.

111. The answer is h. (*Victor, pp 670–671.*) Headaches that occur on standing indicate the presence of intracranial hypotension. Most often, this is the result of recent lumbar puncture, either for diagnostic purposes or after spinal anesthesia. The hole in the dura created by the spinal tap presumably allows fluid to continue leaking out, and this creates a condition of decreased pressure within the spinal canal, which causes traction on the pain-sensitive meninges of the brain. Other causes of intracranial hypotension include continued leak of CSF from the subarachnoid space after head trauma, neurosurgery, or even pneumonectomy (thoracoarachnoid fistula); occult pituitary tumor; a leak from a dural tear in the spinal root sleeves; traumatic nerve root avulsion; or systemic illness such as dehydration, diabetic coma, uremia, or meningoencephalitis. With leakage of CSF into nasal passages, the patient may complain of rhinorrhea. In some cases, no cause is apparent even after a thorough evaluation.

Traumatic and Occupational Injuries

Questions

DIRECTIONS: Each item below contains a question followed by suggested responses. Select the **one best** response to each question.

112. A 35-year-old woman works as a keyboard operator and must type for 6 h per day. She is especially susceptible to injuring which of the following nerves?

a. Axillary nerve
b. Median nerve
c. Ulnar nerve
d. Radial nerve
e. Long thoracic nerve

113. A 28-year-old police officer has been generally healthy except for mild, easily controlled hypertension. He sustains a gunshot wound to the upper arm. This type of trauma may cause partial damage to the median nerve that may leave the patient with which of the following?

a. Easily provoked pain in the hand
b. Weakness on wrist extension
c. Atrophy in the first dorsal interosseous muscle
d. Numbness over the fifth digit
e. Radial deviation of the hand

114. A 19-year-old man is involved in a street fight in which he is viciously attacked with a lead pipe. A particularly forceful blow hits his left elbow. Blunt trauma to the elbow may lead to the development of which of the following?

a. Wristdrop
b. Weakness of the abductor pollicis brevis
c. Clawhand or benediction sign
d. Ulnar deviation of the hand
e. Poor pronation of the forearm

115. A 21-year-old right-handed woman works at an airport as a luggage handler. She is usually on the tarmac working in an environment in which loud noises are routine. Ear protection must be worn to protect against loss of hearing and the development of which of the following?

a. Vertigo
b. Tinnitus
c. Ataxia
d. Diplopia
e. Oscillopsia

116. A young man fractures his humerus in an automobile accident. As the pain from the injury subsides, he notices weakness on attempted flexion at the elbow. He develops paresthesias over the radial and volar aspects of the forearm. During the accident, he probably injured which one of the following nerves?

a. Suprascapular nerve
b. Long thoracic nerve
c. Musculocutaneous nerve
d. Radial nerve
e. Median nerve

117. A 37-year-old alcoholic man awakes with clumsiness of his right hand. Neurologic examination reveals poor extension of the hand at the wrist. He most likely has injured which one of the following nerves?

a. Median nerve
b. Brachioradialis nerve
c. Musculocutaneous nerve
d. Radial nerve
e. Ulnar nerve

118. A 72-year-old man slipped and fell in the bathroom 1 week ago. He hit the right side of his head, but did not think it was necessary to seek medical attention. He finally goes to his doctor because his son thinks his balance is off. Computed tomography (CT) of the brain may fail to reveal a small subdural hematoma in this patient for which of the following reasons?

a. The lesion is subacute
b. The hematoma extends into the brain from the subdural space
c. The resolution of the CT machine is greater than 2 mm
d. The subdural hematoma is less than 4 h old
e. The patient has extensive cerebral atrophy

119. A 16-year-old boy is struck on the side of the head by a bottle thrown by a friend involved in a prank. He appears dazed for about 30 seconds, but is apparently lucid for several minutes before he abruptly becomes stuporous. His limbs on the side opposite the site of the blow are more flaccid than those on the same side as the injury. On arrival in the emergency room 25 minutes after the accident, he is unresponsive to painful stimuli. His pulse is 40/min, with an ECG revealing no arrhythmias. His blood pressure in both arms is 170/110 mmHg. Although papilledema is not evident in his fundi, he has venous distention and absent pulsations of the retinal vasculature. Which of the following is the best explanation for this young man's evolving clinical signs?

a. A seizure disorder
b. A cardiac conduction defect
c. Increased intracranial pressure
d. Sick sinus syndrome
e. Communicating hydrocephalus

120. A 52-year-old patient presents with headache and sudden onset of mania. Her head CT is shown below. Two hours later her blood pressure is 225/110, her heart rate is 40, and her consciousness is fluctuating. Which of the following is the best management over the next 4 h for this patient?

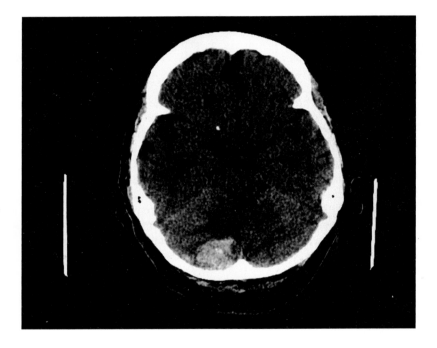

   a. Craniotomy
   b. Antihypertensive medication
   c. Transvenous pacemaker placement
   d. Ventriculoperitoneal shunt
   e. Antiepileptic medication

121. A 64-year-old woman slips and falls on an icy sidewalk. She hits the side of her head on the curb. After a momentary loss of consciousness she recovers, but is in some pain. Fifteen minutes later her level of consciousness begins to fluctuate and she is brought to the emergency room comatose. Magnetic resonance imaging (MRI) of the patient's head within the first few hours of injury should reveal which of the following?

a. A normal brain
b. Intracerebral hematoma
c. Temporal lobe contusion
d. Subarachnoid hemorrhage
e. Epidural hematoma

122. Computed tomography scanning of a patient's head within 2 hours of a newly acquired epidural hematoma should reveal which of the following?

a. A normal brain
b. A lens-shaped density over the frontal lobe
c. Increased CSF density with a fluid-fluid level
d. Multifocal attenuation of cortical tissue
e. Bilateral sickle-shaped densities over the hemispheres

123. The elderly person who suffers relatively mild head trauma but who subsequently develops a progressive dementia over the course of several weeks is most likely to have sustained which of the following?

a. An acute subdural hematoma
b. An acute epidural hematoma
c. A chronic subdural hematoma
d. An intracerebral hematoma
e. An intracerebellar hematoma

124. A 42-year-old woman is involved in a head-on collision with a lamppost at 50 mph. Her head hits the windshield. She is highly likely to have an intracranial hemorrhage in which one of the following structures?

a. Occipital lobe
b. Thalamus
c. Putamen
d. Parietal lobe
e. Temporal lobe

125. A 57-year-old woman is involved in a motor vehicle accident in which she strikes the windshield and is briefly unconscious. She makes a full recovery, except that 3 months later she notices that she cannot taste the food she is eating. This is most likely due to which of the following?

a. Medullary infarction
b. Temporal lobe contusion
c. Sphenoid sinus hemorrhage
d. Phenytoin use to prevent seizures
e. Avulsion of olfactory rootlets

126. An 18-year-old boy is brought into the emergency room after a diving accident. He is awake and alert, has intact cranial nerves, and is able to move his shoulders, but he cannot move his arms or legs. He is flaccid and has a sensory level at C5. Appropriate management includes which of the following?

a. Naloxone hydrochloride
b. Intravenous methylprednisolone
c. Oral dexamethasone
d. Phenytoin 100 mg tid
e. Hyperbaric oxygen therapy

Traumatic and Occupational Injuries

Answers

112. The answer is b. (*Victor, pp 1433–1434.*) Pressure on the volar aspect of the wrist may produce recurrent injuries to the carpal tunnel through which the median nerve runs. The injury characteristically produces pain and paresthesias in the hand over the distribution of the sensory component of the median nerve. This sensory distribution extends over the palmar surface of the thumb and first four digits, with the fourth digit supplied on one side by the median nerve and on the other side by the ulnar nerve. Median nerve injuries are consequently said to split the fourth digit on sensory examinations. With carpal tunnel compression of the median nerve, the sensory disturbance may be incapacitating. Subsequently, weakness and atrophy may develop in the muscles that are innervated by the median nerve. The abductor pollicis brevis may be severely involved late in the progression of the disorder.

113. The answer is a. (*Victor, pp 1438–1439.*) Trauma to nerves in the extremities may give rise to causalgia, a disturbance in sensory perception characterized by hypesthesia, dysesthesia, and allodynia. Hypesthesia is a decrease in the accurate perception of stimuli. Dysesthesia is persistent discomfort, which in the situation described is likely to be an unremitting burning pain. Allodynia is the perception of pain with the application of nonpainful stimuli. Bullets and other high-velocity missiles need not hit the nerve to cause damage. Enough energy is transmitted as the missile passes through adjacent tissues to produce substantial damage to the nerve. Choices **b** through **d** involve motor or sensory findings due to either ulnar or radial nerve damage.

114. The answer is c. (*Victor, p 1434.*) The ulnar nerve runs superficially at the elbow in the ulnar groove. It continues forward under the aponeurosis of the flexor carpi ulnaris in the cubital tunnel. Damage to the nerve at this site may produce weakness in the interosseous and ulnar lumbrical muscles of the hand. With lumbrical weakness, the extensor sheaths of the digits are not properly positioned, and a claw deformity with impaired extension of the ulnar two digits develops when the patient tries to straighten his or her fingers.

115. The answer is b. (*Victor, pp 308–309.*) Acoustic trauma may produce severe tinnitus in persons who have relatively little hearing loss. Although the initial injury with acoustic trauma is sustained by the cochlear sensory cells, tinnitus may persist even after the acoustic nerve is cut. Tinnitus may take any one of several forms, ranging from a hissing sound to a high-pitched screaming noise.

116. The answer is c. (*Victor, p 1432.*) The musculocutaneous nerve is often damaged with fractures of the humerus. This nerve supplies the biceps brachii, brachialis, and coracobrachialis muscles and carries sensory information from the lateral cutaneous nerve of the forearm. Flexion at the elbow with damage to this nerve is most impaired with the forearm supinated.

117. The answer is d. (*Victor, pp 1432–1433.*) Radial nerve injuries are fairly common in alcoholic persons who may have lost consciousness in awkward positions. These are sometimes referred to as Saturday night palsies. The injury is usually a pressure palsy and produces a wristdrop. The nerve is injured as it courses near the spiral groove of the humerus.

118. The answer is a. (*Lee, pp 440–444.*) Within a few days of formation, the contents of a subdural hematoma are degraded into less dense fluid. This fluid is transiently similar in density to the cerebral cortex. If the fluid collection is too small to produce substantial deformation of the underlying hemisphere, identification of the subdural collection may be difficult. Angiogram will reveal displacement of the cerebrocortical vessels, but more rapid and less invasive assessment of the patient is feasible with MRI.

119. The answer is c. (*Victor, pp 948–950.*) Something has abruptly caused increasing intracranial pressure in this young man after his head trauma. Consequently, he is at risk for herniation of the brain transfalcially (across the falx cerebri) or transtentorially (across the tentorium cerebelli). The head trauma produced an intracranial lesion, which is expanding very rapidly. The slowing of his pulse and increase in his blood pressure are due to the Cushing effect of a rapidly expanding intracranial mass.

120. The answer is a. *(Victor, p 888.)* Without emergency surgery, the patient will die. Her blood pressure and pulse abnormalities will correct themselves when the intracranial mass is removed. Her loss of consciousness will not correct itself with antiepileptics. Shunt placement will not likely prevent brain herniation and may in fact accelerate it. The hematoma must be evacuated, and the bleeding giving rise to the hematoma must be stopped.

121. The answer is e. *(Victor, pp 937–938.)* The history is typical for an epidural hematoma. Damage to the middle meningeal artery allows blood at arterial pressures to dissect in the potential space that exists between the dura mater and the periosteum of the skull. With MRI, the epidural hematoma should be evident soon after the injury, and will certainly be evident by the time the patient is symptomatic.

122. The answer is b. *(Victor, pp 937–938.)* The typical shape of an epidural hematoma is that of a biconvex mass that displaces normal brain tissue. Parts of the ventricular system may be dilated as obstructive hydrocephalus develops in parts of the system. Transfalcial herniation with displacement of frontal lobe tissue across the midline and under the falx cerebri is likely with an epidural hematoma on one side of the head. Although subdural hematomas are often bilateral, epidural hematomas are invariably unilateral.

123. The answer is c. *(Victor, p 452.)* Chronic subdural hematoma is relatively common in the elderly and in patients receiving renal dialysis. The subdural fluid becomes isodense with the brain after several days or weeks and may be overlooked on CT scanning. Magnetic resonance imaging will identify the lesion, even if it is present bilaterally and produces no shift of brain structures from the midline.

124. The answer is e. *(Bradley, p 1130.)* The temporal lobes and inferior frontal lobes are frequently involved in traumatic brain injuries. The continued forward movement of the brain within the bony cranial vault, which has suddenly decelerated at impact, leads to these anterior brain structures striking the inside of the skull with great force, creating contusions in these areas. The rough surfaces of the cribriform plate and the middle cranial fossa also lead to injury in these locations. These injuries are referred to as the *coup injuries* because they reflect the direct blow to the brain. So-called contrecoup injury may also occur at the diametrically opposed region of the brain (generally, the occipital lobes) when there is rebound movement into the overlying skull there. Damage to the temporal lobe may produce symptoms and signs by virtue of compression of adjacent brain structures. As a hematoma expands, uncal herniation may crush the brainstem. Less progressive injuries may disturb memory or even language comprehension. Wernicke's area, which is important in language comprehension, is sufficiently posterior on the temporal lobe to escape injury in most cases of frontal head trauma.

125. The answer is e. (*Victor, pp 927–928.*) Anosmia is one of the more common long-term cranial nerve deficits after head injury, though it is present in only 6% in one series. It is often associated with ageusia (loss of taste). It can be very disabling and discouraging to patients. Approximately one-third of patients recover. It is caused by avulsion of olfactory nerve rootlets due to acceleration-deceleration injury at the cribriform plate. Damage may be unilateral or bilateral.

126. The answer is b. (*Victor, pp 1300–1301.*) High-dose intravenous methylprednisolone [30-mg/kg intravenous bolus followed by 5.4 mg/(kg·h) for 23 h] has been shown to have a statistically significant, if clinically modest, benefit on the outcome after spinal cord injury when given within 8 h of the injury. Naloxone hydrochloride and other agents, such as G_{M1} ganglioside, have not been shown to be of benefit. The role of surgical decompression, removal of hemorrhage, and correction of bone displacement is controversial. Most American neurosurgeons do not advocate surgery, and instead propose external spinal fixation.

Infections

Questions

DIRECTIONS: Each item below contains a question followed by suggested responses. Select the **one best** response to each question.

127. The most striking neurologic complication of von Economo's encephalitis (encephalitis lethargica), a type of encephalitis that occurred in epidemic proportions along with viral influenza between 1917 and 1928, was which of the following?

a. Blindness
b. Hearing loss
c. Paraplegia
d. Parkinsonism
e. Incontinence

128. A 37-year-old woman is noted to have lymphadenopathy on routine physical exam. Following an extensive evaluation, she is diagnosed with sarcoid. She has been entirely normal neurologically. Which cranial nerve is most likely to be injured in this patient?

a. II
b. III
c. V
d. VII
e. VIII

129. A 17-year-old female presents initially with fever and progressive weakness. An extensive neurological evaluation including EMG/NCS suggests a motor neuron disease. The motor neuron disease most certainly traced to a virus is which of the following?

a. Poliomyelitis
b. Subacute sclerosing panencephalitis (SSPE)
c. Progressive multifocal leukoencephalopathy (PML)
d. Subacute HIV encephalomyelitis
e. Kuru

130. A 35-year-old woman who has received a liver transplant develops meningeal signs and fever. Cerebrospinal fluid testing reveals a fungal infection. Which of the following is the most common cause of fungal meningitis?

a. *Aspergillus*
b. *Candida*
c. *Mucor*
d. *Cryptococcus*
e. *Rhizopus*

131. A 28-year-old man who has recently immigrated from Brazil presents with 3 months of fluctuating but slowly progressive bilateral lower extremity weakness, a little worse on the left side than on the right. After a complete evaluation, *Schistosoma mansoni* is diagnosed as the etiology. *S. mansoni* ova usually damage the nervous system at the level of which of the following?

a. Cerebrum
b. Cerebellum
c. Basal ganglia
d. Spinal cord
e. Peripheral nerves

132. A 12-year-old boy has left body weakness. An brain MRI scan reveals a polycystic lesion. The parasitic brain lesion most likely to have a large cyst containing numerous daughter cysts is that associated with which of the following?

a. *Taenia solium*
b. *Schistosoma haematobium*
c. *Taenia echinococcus*
d. *Diphyllobothrium latum*
e. *Schistosoma japonicum*

133. An 82-year-old previously healthy woman with a recent upper respiratory infection presents with generalized weakness, headache, and blurry vision. For the past 2 weeks she has had upper respiratory symptoms that started with a sore throat, nasal congestion, and excessive coughing. She went to her primary care doctor 4 days ago and was diagnosed with sinusitis. She was given a prescription for an antibiotic and took it for 2 days, then stopped. She thereafter had chills, lightheadedness, vomiting, blurry vision, general achiness, and a headache that started abruptly and has not gotten better since. Except for blurry vision, she has not had any other visual symptoms. The blurry vision remains when she closes either eye. She also has eye tenderness with movement and mild photosensitivity. She has no drug allergies. Exam findings include temperature of 102.5°F, nuchal rigidity, and sleepiness. Which of the following is the next most appropriate action in this case?

a. Get a brain MRI, then perform a lumbar puncture
b. Give the patient a prescription for oral azithromycin and let her go home
c. Immediately give intravenous ceftriaxone plus ampicillin
d. Immediately start intravenous acyclovir
e. Obtain cerebrospinal fluid and blood cultures and observe the patient until the results come back

134. Routine spinal fluid examination in a patient with spongiform encephalopathy would be expected to show which of the following?

a. No abnormalities on routine studies
b. Elevated protein
c. More than 100 lymphocytes
d. More than 1000 red blood cells
e. Decreased glucose

135. A 17-year-old right-handed boy has had infectious meningitis 8 times over the past 3 years. He has otherwise been generally healthy and developed normally. Recurrent meningitis often develops in persons with which of the following?

a. Otitis media
b. Epilepsy
c. Multiple sclerosis
d. Whipple's disease
e. Cerebrospinal fluid (CSF) leaks

136. An 82-year-old man with a history of pulmonary tuberculosis in 1947 presents with left body weakness and neglect. Imaging and subsequent biopsy reveal that recurrent tuberculosis was the cause. Mass lesions in the brain of the patient with tuberculosis may develop as a reaction to the tubercle bacillus and consist of which of the following?

a. Dysplastic central nervous system (CNS) tissue
b. Caseating granulomas
c. Heterotopias
d. Colobomas
e. Mesial sclerosis

137. A 31-year-old homosexual man has had headache, sleepiness, and poor balance that have worsened over the past week. The patient is known to be HIV-seropositive, but has done well in the past and has not seen a doctor in over 1 year. On examination, his responses are slow and he has some difficulty sustaining attention. He has a right hemiparesis with increased reflexes on the right. Routine cell counts and chemistries are normal. Which of the following is the most appropriate next step in management?

a. Head CT with contrast
b. Noncontrast head CT
c. Perform a lumbar puncture
d. Start antiretroviral therapy
e. Start intravenous heparin

138. A 52-year-old woman with AIDS presents to the emergency room with mild left hemiparesis and altered mental status. A CT scan reveals several rim-enhancing lesions with minimal mass effect. Which of the following is the best next step in management?

a. Get a cerebral angiogram
b. Order a ventricular cerebrospinal fluid (CSF) aspiration
c. Perform a lumbar puncture and include cerebrospinal fluid for Epstein-Barr virus (EBV) PCR in tests ordered
d. Stop all antiretroviral therapy
e. Treat with intravenous acyclovir

139. A 32-year-old intravenous drug abuser presents with more than 2 weeks of left body weakness. Brain CT scan reveals several ring-enhancing lesions, and an HIV test is positive. Serological, CSF, and MRI testing support the diagnosis of *Toxoplasma gondii*. Which of the following is the best treatment for HIV associated CNS *Toxoplasma gondii*?

a. Intravenous acyclovir
b. Neurosurgical removal of the lesions
c. Oral fluconazole
d. Sulfadiazine and pyrimethamine
e. Thiabendazole

140. A 35-year-old female has progressive numbness of the right arm and difficulty seeing objects in the left visual field. She is known to be HIV-positive, but has not consistently taken medications in the past. On examination, she appears healthy, but has a right homonymous hemianopsia and decreased sensory perception in her left upper extremity and face. Her CD4 count is 75 cells per µL, and her MRI is consistent with a demylinating lesion of the left parietooccipital area. CSF PCR for JC virus is positive. Which of the following is the most appropriate treatment in this case?

a. Amphotericin B
b. Cranial radiation
c. Highly active antiretroviral therapy (HAART)
d. Intravenous acyclovir
e. Intravenous ceftriaxone

141. A 72-year-old right-handed woman has 2 days of headache and fever, followed by worsening confusion. She is taken to the hospital after having a generalized seizure. A head CT is consistent with left temporal hemorrhage and swelling. Localization of an encephalitis to the medial temporal or orbital frontal regions of the brain is most consistent with which of the following?

a. *Treponema pallidum*
b. Varicella zoster virus
c. Herpes simplex virus
d. *Cryptococcus neoformans*
e. *Toxoplasma gondii*

142. A 21-year-old college student was found walking around his dormitory naked. He is disoriented, inattentive, and shows poor comprehension. In the emergency room he is found to have a fever of 102°F. There are no apparent motor, sensory, or coordination abnormalities. The emergency room physician orders a brain MRI and then decides to perform a lumbar puncture. Neuroimaging of the brain before attempting a lumbar puncture is advisable in cases of acute encephalitis for which one of the following reasons?

a. The diagnosis may be evident on the basis of magnetic resonance imaging (MRI) alone
b. Massive edema in the temporal lobe may make herniation imminent
c. The computed tomography (CT) picture may determine whether a brain biopsy should be obtained
d. Shunting of the ventricles is usually indicated, and the imaging studies are needed to direct the placement of the shunt
e. It may establish which pathology is responsible

143. A 67-year-old man presents with headache, fever, disorientation, and seizures. CSF testing establishes that the patient has the most common form of acute encephalitis. The CSF changes late in the course of this disease typically include which of the following?

a. An increased number of lymphocytes
b. A glucose content of less than two-thirds the serum level
c. A protein content of less than 45 mg/dL
d. A normal opening pressure
e. A predominance of polymorphonuclear white blood cells

144. A 27-year-old man presents to his primary care doctor with a low-grade fever, headache, and neck stiffness, which have become more bothersome over the past 1 to 2 weeks. CSF and serological testing for Lyme is positive and antibiotic treatment is initiated. The cranial neuropathy most commonly found with Lyme disease is that associated with damage to which cranial nerve?

a. III
b. V
c. VII
d. IX
e. XII

145. The pathologic specimen depicted here shows the only intracranial lesion found in this patient. This patient would be expected to have exhibited which of the following symptoms?

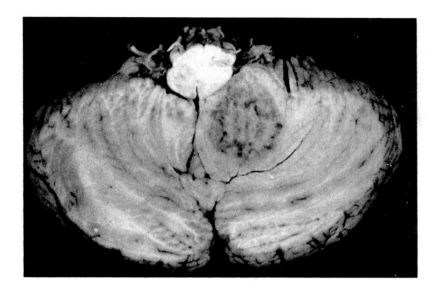

a. Seizures
b. Gait ataxia
c. Hemiparesis
d. Visual loss
e. Hallucinations

146. A 13-year-old boy is brought into the emergency room lethargic with a stiff neck and fever. Despite aggressive therapy, the child dies. Postmortem evaluation reveals that the child had primary amebic meningoencephalitis. This condition is usually acquired through which of the following means?

a. Freshwater swimming
b. Eating contaminated meat
c. Eating calves' brains
d. Anal intercourse
e. Animal bites

147. Both HIV and cytomegalovirus infections in the brain characteristically produce which of the following?

a. Senile plaques
b. Intraneuronal amyloid
c. Intranuclear inclusions
d. Intracytoplasmic inclusions
e. Microglial nodules

148. Following several days of low-grade fever and mild neck and head pain, a 10-year-old boy develops bilateral face drooping and difficulty fully closing his eyes. Serum is positive for *Borrelia burgdorferi* IgM. CSF PCR is also positive for this organism's DNA. After *B. burgdorferi* is introduced by the tick that carries it, the skin around the bite develops which of the following?

a. An exfoliative dermatitis
b. Purpura
c. Localized edema
d. Erythema chronicum migrans
e. Vesicular lesions

149. A 59-year-old right-handed woman has been clinically diagnosed with encephalitis. While CSF and MRI studies are pending, a medical student suggests ordering an EEG. Which of the following EEG findings is most associated with herpes encephalitis?

a. α activity over the frontal regions
b. β activity over the temporal regions
c. Three-per-second spike-and-wave discharges
d. Bilateral, periodic epileptiform discharges
e. Unilateral δ activity over the frontal region

150. Which of the following medications is most appropriate in patients with CNS involvement by *B. burgdorferi*?

a. Streptomycin
b. Ceftriaxone
c. Gentamicin
d. Isoniazid
e. Rifampin

151. A 41-year-old homosexual man is brought to medical attention by his partner because of headache, sluggish mentation, and impaired ambulation worsening over the previous week. The patient is known to be HIV-seropositive, but has done well in the past and has not sought regular medical attention. On examination, his responses are slow and he has some difficulty sustaining attention. He has a right hemiparesis with increased reflexes on the right. Routine cell counts and chemistries are normal. A contrast head CT reveals several ring-enhancing lesions. Eventually, surgical aspiration of one of the lesions reveals that they are abscesses. Abscesses in the brain most often develop from which of the following?

a. Hematogenous spread of infection
b. Penetrating head wounds
c. Superinfection of neoplastic foci
d. Dental trauma
e. Neurosurgical intervention

152. Which of the following is the most common site for abscess formation in the brain?

a. Putamen
b. Thalamus
c. Head of the caudate
d. Gray-white junction
e. Subthalamus

153. An 8-year-old girl is bitten on her hand while feeding a wild raccoon. Her parents have many questions regarding diseases that she may have contracted. Which of the following is the best therapy currently available for rabies?

a. Supportive therapy
b. Zidovudine
c. Cytarabine
d. Amantadine
e. Ganciclovir

154. Which of the following consequences of disseminated syphilis may present a picture easily confused with brain tumor?

a. A reaction to penicillin treatment occurs
b. An intracranial gumma forms
c. Tabes dorsalis is the primary manifestation of the disease
d. Meningovascular syphilis develops
e. The patient is a newborn with congenital syphilis

155. From the brain, rabies virus establishes itself for transmission to another host by spreading to which of the following?

a. Intestines
b. Nasopharynx
c. Lungs
d. Bladder
e. Salivary glands

156. A 38-year-old man who is immunocompromised because of HIV presents with 1 month of worsening right headache, ear pain, and fever. He is determined to have malignant external otitis and osteomyelitis of the base of the skull. The etiology is fungal. Fungal malignant external otitis and osteomyelitis of the base of the skull in HIV patients is most commonly caused by which of the following?

a. *Nocardia*
b. *Cryptococcus neoformans*
c. *Actinomyces*
d. *Aspergillus*
e. *Candida*

157. A 55-year-old woman has progressive dementia over the past year. Over the past 3 months she has also developed dysarthria, myoclonus, intention tremor, and hyperreflexia. CSF VDRL is positive. This patient's symptoms are being caused by which of the following?

a. A response to penicillin treatment
b. An autoimmune reaction
c. An acute meningoencephalitis
d. A chronic meningoencephalitis
e. A chronic rhombencephalitis

158. Which of the following is the most common cause of brain abscess in patients with AIDS?

a. *Cryptococcus neoformans*
b. *Toxoplasma gondii*
c. Tuberculosis
d. Cytomegalovirus
e. Herpes zoster

159. A 35-year-old woman is bitten by a small doglike wild animal while camping. The animal immediately runs away. Her skin is barely broken, and, besides feeling a little frightened, she says that she is fine. Despite this, her friend convinces her to be evaluated in the nearest emergency room. Which of the following viruses that typically invade the CNS by extending centripetally (i.e., inward away from the periphery) along peripheral nerves is the woman most at risk for?

a. Mumps
b. Measles
c. Varicella zoster
d. Polio
e. Rabies

160. Which of the following is the most common symptom in patients with brain abscess?

a. Nausea and vomiting
b. Ataxia
c. Headache
d. Neck stiffness
e. Seizures

161. Most of the organisms found in brain abscesses are which of the following?

a. Streptococcal
b. Staphylococcal
c. *Bacteroides* spp.
d. *Proteus* spp.
e. *Pseudomonas* spp.

162. A 52-year-old woman develops progressive dementia, tremors, gait ataxia, and myoclonic jerks over the course of 6 months. Her speech is slow and slurred, and hand movements are clumsy. No members of her immediate family have a history of degenerative neurologic disease. Magnetic resonance imaging (MRI) of the head reveals a subtle increase in T2 signal in the basal ganglia bilaterally. EEG reveals disorganized background activity with periodic sharp-wave discharges that occur repetitively at 1-s intervals and extend over both sides of the head. Arteriogram reveals no vascular abnormalities. The clinical picture is most consistent with which of the following?

a.   Multi-infarct dementia
b.   Tabes dorsalis
c.   Friedreich's disease (Friedreich's ataxia)
d.   Subarachnoid hemorrhage
e.   Spongiform encephalopathy

163. Which of the following is the drug of choice for treating a 75-year-old with *Listeria monocytogenes* meningitis?

a.   Penicillin G
b.   Ampicillin plus gentamicin
c.   Tetracycline
d.   Ceftriaxone
e.   Rifampin

164. A patient with an 8-month history of neurological decline dies after a severe bout of aspiration pneumonia. Autopsy of her brain reveals extensive loss of granule cells in the cerebellum and other changes most obvious in the cerebellar cortex. Fine vacuoles give the brain a spongiform appearance. No senile plaques are evident. The patient could have acquired this progressive disease through which of the following means?

a.   Sexual intercourse
b.   A blood transfusion
c.   Consumption of raw fish
d.   An upper respiratory infection
e.   Growth hormone treatment

DIRECTIONS: Each group of questions below consists of lettered options followed by a set of numbered items. For each numbered item, select the **one** lettered option with which it is **most** closely associated. Each lettered option may be used once, more than once, or not at all.

Questions 165–170

Select the condition that best fits each clinical scenario.

a. Subacute HIV encephalomyelitis (AIDS encephalopathy)
b. Subacute sclerosing panencephalitis (SSPE)
c. Progressive multifocal leukoencephalopathy (PML)
d. Rabies encephalitis
e. Guillain-Barré syndrome
f. Tabes dorsalis
g. Neurocysticercosis
h. *Bartonella henselae* encephalitis
i. HTLV-I infection

165. A 27-year-old man develops recurrent episodes of involuntary movements. He abused intravenous drugs for several years and has had several admissions for recurrent infections, including subacute bacterial endocarditis. His involuntary movements are largely restricted to the right side of his body and are associated with hoarseness and difficulty swallowing. The patient has lost 40 lb over the past 4 months. Examination reveals diffuse lymphadenopathy and right-sided hypertonia. His CSF is normal except for a slight increase in protein content. Computed tomography reveals a large area of decreased density on the left side of the cerebrum. EEG reveals diffuse slowing over the left side of the head. Biopsy of this lesion reveals oligodendrocytes with abnormally large nuclei that contain darkly staining inclusions. There is extensive demyelination and there are giant astrocytes in the lesion. Over the course of 1 month, the man exhibits increasing ataxia. Within 2 months, he shows evidence of mild dementia and seizures. Within 3 months of presentation, his dementia is profound and he has bladder and bowel incontinence. Over the course of a few days, he becomes obtunded and dies.

166. An 18-year-old man notices tingling about his ankles 2 weeks after an upper respiratory tract infection. Within 2 days, he has weakness in dorsiflexion of both feet, and within 1 week he develops problems with walking. He has no loss of bladder or bowel control. His weakness progresses rapidly over the ensuing week and necessitates his being placed on a ventilator to support his breathing. He is quadriplegic, but retains control of his eye movements. Cerebrospinal fluid studies reveal a protein content of greater than 1 g/dL with a normal white cell count. There are no red blood cells in the CSF.

167. Over the course of 6 months, a 50-year-old immigrant from Eastern Europe develops problems with bladder control, an unsteady gait, and pain in his legs. On examination, it is determined that he has absent deep tendon reflexes in his legs, markedly impaired vibration sense in his feet, and a positive Romberg sign. Despite his complaint of unsteady gait, he has no problems with rapid alternating movement of the feet and no tremors are evident. He has normal leg strength. The pain in his legs is sharp, stabbing, and paroxysmal. His serum glucose and glycohemoglobin levels are normal.

168. A 10-year-old girl is referred to a physician because of rapidly deteriorating school performance. Over the course of a few weeks, the child has lost interest in her schoolwork, appeared apathetic at home, and had frequent temper tantrums with little provocation. A psychiatric evaluation reveals that, in addition to emotional lability, the child has substantial intellectual deficits that appear to be new. Within 1 month of this evaluation, the child has a generalized tonic-clonic seizure. A neurologist examining the child discovers chorioretinitis, ataxia, hyperactive reflexes, and bilateral Babinski signs. Her EEG exhibits periodic bursts of high-voltage slow waves followed by recurrent low-voltage stretches (burst suppression pattern). The CSF is remarkable for an increase in the gamma globulin fraction. The child becomes increasingly lethargic and obtunded over the ensuing 2 months. She remains in a coma for several months before dying.

169. A 37-year-old female Navy officer presents with 3 days of confusion and seizures. Her colleagues report that she has been acting strangely for 3 days. This is followed by generalized status epilepticus. The woman has previously been well. She has traveled to the Caribbean several times annually, and she has a new pet cat. General exam discloses epitrochlear lymphadenopathy. Neurologic exam shows the woman to be in status epilepticus. Cerebrospinal fluid is negative; MRI shows increased signal in the pulvinar bilaterally.

170. A 29-year-old immigrant from El Salvador is brought to the emergency room after a generalized seizure. After awakening, he relates that he has had two or three episodes of unexplained loss of consciousness in the past 2 years. He has otherwise been healthy. He served in the Salvadoran military for 3 years. His examination is normal. Computed tomography scan with contrast reveals two small hyperintense foci in the right frontal lobe, as well as a 1-cm cystic lesion with a nodular focus within it in the left frontal region. The cyst wall of the latter lesion enhances with contrast. The two right frontal lesions do not enhance.

Infections

Answers

127. The answer is d. (*Victor, p 813.*) At the onset of encephalitis lethargica, patients often develop transient fevers, lethargy, and headache. Disturbed eye movements are the most common sign of neurologic disease during the acute illness. A variety of movement disorders, including chorea, athetosis, dystonia, and myoclonus, develop with the disease. About one in four affected persons dies. The most common sequela of the disease is severe, unremitting parkinsonism with signs and symptoms similar to those exhibited with idiopathic parkinsonism (paralysis agitans). One rather unique feature is the occurrence of oculogyric crises, or episodes in which the eyes deviate to one side or upward, associated with other forms of dystonia and autonomic symptoms, sometimes occurring with great regularity.

128. The answer is d. (*Bradley, p 2375.*) Facial paresis is the neurologic injury most likely to develop with sarcoidosis. Almost half of patients with sarcoidosis and neurologic disease have a neurologic sign or symptom as the first obvious complication of the sarcoidosis. These patients report progressive weakness of one side of the face with no substantial loss of sensation over the paretic side. They may feel that there is decreased sensitivity to touch on the weak side, but this is more commonly from a loss of tone in the facial muscles than from an injury to the trigeminal nerve. Other cranial nerves especially susceptible to injury in persons with sarcoidosis include II, III, IV, VI, and VIII.

129. The answer is a. (*Bradley, pp 2231–2232.*) SSPE, PML, kuru, and HIV encephalomyelitis are all viral diseases affecting the CNS, but poliomyelitis is the only one that causes a purely motor neuron disease. Poliomyelitis virus attacks the anterior horn cells in the spinal cord. It is most likely to be confused with Guillain-Barré syndrome if the typical CSF picture of a viral meningoencephalitis is not found with the progressive motor neuron impairment. With poliomyelitis, the CSF will usually exhibit an elevated protein and white cell count. During the initial stages of the infection, the patient will usually have fever.

130. The answer is d. (*Bradley, p 1546.*) Cryptococcosis is usually acquired through the lungs and spreads to the CNS through the bloodstream. In the CNS, it may produce either a meningitis or a meningoencephalitis. The organism has a characteristic capsule, which simplifies its identification. Fungal infections most often occur in the CNS in persons with defects in their immune systems. These defects may be secondary to a viral infection, as with AIDS, or they may be a consequence of immunosuppressive drug exposure. Patients on immunosuppressive treatment after organ transplants and those with lymphoproliferative disorders, such as lymphocytic leukemia, were the most common victims of CNS fungal infections before the start of the AIDS epidemic. *Aspergillus, Candida, Mucor,* and *Rhizopus* can also cause CNS fungal infections, but rarely meningitis. *Aspergillus* tends to cause abscesses in immunocompromised individuals, and *Mucor* affects mostly diabetics.

131. The answer is d. (*Bradley, pp 1576–1577.*) *S. mansoni* is endemic in Puerto Rico and may produce a subacutely evolving paraparesis. The fluke itself does not invade the spinal cord, but it deposits eggs in the valveless veins of Batson, which drain the intestines and communicate with the drainage from the lumbosacral spinal cord. The patient develops granulomas around the ova that lodge in the spinal cord, and these granulomatous lesions crush the cord.

132. The answer is c. (*Bradley, p 1573.*) Echinococcosis is usually acquired by eating tissue from infected sheep. Children are more likely to develop cerebral lesions than adults, but people at any age may develop this encephalic hydatidosis, which entails the development of a major cyst with multiple compartments in which smaller cysts are evident. This hydatid cyst of the brain behaves like a tumor and may become massive enough to cause focal deficits.

133. The answer is c. (*Bradley, pp 1476–1483.*) The immediate concern is that the patient has bacterial meningitis, and she should be treated. A lumbar puncture and blood draw to obtain cultures should be done; however, it can take a few days for the results to come back, and it may be too late for the patient by then. Oral azithromycin is not the proper treatment for bacterial meningitis. Intravenous acyclovir would be used to treat herpes encephalitis.

134. The answer is a. *(Bradley, p 1624.)* The spinal fluid examination in a patient with spongiform encephalopathy, or Creutzfeldt-Jakob disease, is typically normal. On occasion, the protein level may be mildly elevated, and, in up to 20% of cases, there may be an increase in the ratio of immunoglobulin G to total protein, occasionally with oligoclonal bands. Studies have indicated that a protein highly sensitive and specific for prion disease, a 14-3-3 proteinase inhibitor protein released from neurons, may be found in patients with this illness.

135. The answer is e. *(Victor, pp 788–790.)* A CSF leak indicates a communication between the subarachnoid space and the surface of the body. This leak most often occurs through the nose as rhinorrhea or through the ear as otorrhea. The CSF may be distinguished from other fluid discharged from the nose or ear by its relatively obvious glucose content. The most common basis for a CSF leak is head trauma.

136. The answer is b. *(Victor, p 759.)* Rupture of a large caseating granuloma into the ventricles or the subarachnoid space may produce an abrupt and often lethal deterioration. If the mass becomes large enough before it ruptures, it may in all respects imitate a brain tumor. Such lesions may respond to antituberculous medications even when they are quite large, and the patient may be spared surgical intervention.

137. The answer is a. *(Victor, pp 12–19.)* The differential diagnosis is rather broad at this point. One should look for an infectious or malignant mass with a contrast-enhanced CT or MRI. A noncontrast head CT is less sensitive for abscess or tumor. A lumbar puncture should be done only after you are sure that there is not significant mass effect. This patient has an acute problem, which should be addressed now. Antiretroviral therapy will help him in the long term, but does not need to be initiated in the emergency room. Intravenous heparin is a treatment for embolic stroke. Embolic stroke is unlikely in this case, and further evaluation is needed before treatment with intravenous heparin is considered.

138. The answer is c. *(Bradley, pp 1592–1596.)* The most common etiologies of rim-enhancing brain lesions in AIDS patients are primary CNS lymphoma (PCNSL) and *Toxoplasma gondii* infection. Other etiologies such as bacterial or fungal abscess are also possible. CSF EBV PCR test is highly sensitive and specific for PCNSL. Since there is no mass effect, it is safe to do a lumbar puncture, so a ventricular cerebrospinal fluid (CSF) aspiration is not necessary. A cerebral angiogram should be done if you suspect an aneurysm or vascular malformation. These are unlikely in this case. There is no reason to stop all antiretroviral therapy. Intravenous acyclovir is used to treat herpes encephalitis, which is unlikely in this case.

139. The answer is d. *(Bradley, pp 1593–1594.)* Sulfadiazine and pyrimethamine is proper treatment for *T. gondii* infection. Neurosurgical removal of the lesions is not indicated. Oral fluconazole is a treatment for fungal infections. Intravenous acyclovir is used to treat herpes encephalitis. Thiabendazole is used to treat helminth infections.

140. The answer is c. *(Bradley, pp 1594–1596.)* The patient has progressive multifocal leukoencephalopathy. It is caused by the JC virus, which is a double-stranded DNA virus. The prognosis is poor, but HAART has been known to be effective in improving survival. JC virus is ubiquitous and may be transmitted through respiratory secretions. Cranial radiation is used to treat malignancies. Amphotericin B is used to treat fungal infections. Intravenous acyclovir is not effective against JC virus, but is used to treat herpes simplex virus encephalitis. Intravenous ceftriaxone is used to treat bacterial meningitis.

141. The answer is c. *(Victor, pp 793–795.)* Herpes simplex type 1 is the strain usually responsible for a herpetic encephalitis. Type 2 may occur in newborns who have been exposed during passage through the birth canal of a woman with genital herpes. Persons with AIDS are also at risk for either type 1 or type 2. Temporal lobe involvement in the immunocompetent patient may produce unilateral swelling and hemorrhage into the temporal lobe.

142. The answer is b. *(Victor, pp 793–795.)* Although there is some controversy regarding whether lumbar puncture can precipitate herniation with a herpes encephalitis, most authorities believe it is best to assess the risk of herniation before doing a lumbar puncture. Cerebrospinal fluid examination is vital in establishing the diagnosis. A variety of infections may mimic herpes in both course and anatomic distribution. The CSF cultures and analysis of CSF constituents help to establish the probable cause of the encephalitis and to direct therapy.

143. The answer is a. (*Victor, pp 793–795.*) The increased number of lymphocytes in the CSF of the patient with herpes encephalitis ranges from more than 12 to several hundred cells per cubic millimeter of fluid. Red blood cells may be apparent in the CSF late in the course of the disease, but their absence does not eliminate the possibility of herpes encephalitis. Cerebrospinal fluid pressure is usually increased, and the glucose content is usually normal or only slightly depressed.

144. The answer is c. (*Victor, pp 768–770.*) Facial weakness may be the only neurologic sign of Lyme disease. The neurologic deficits usually appear weeks after the initial rash. Untreated neurologic disease may persist for months. The facial palsy or optic neuritis that develops with CNS disease is characteristically associated with meningitis.

145. The answer is b. (*Bradley, pp 2169–2171.*) This specimen is a transverse section through the brainstem and cerebellum. There is a large area of discoloration and disturbed anatomy in the left cerebellar hemisphere that is producing little mass effect. Because this is the only lesion postulated for this patient, there is no reason to suspect seizure activity, because that phenomenon would be unlikely in the absence of a cerebrocortical (or at least cerebral) lesion. The other findings listed would similarly not be expected in a patient with cerebellar damage.

146. The answer is a. (*Bradley, pp 1564–1566.*) Primary amebic meningoencephalitis is usually caused by organisms from the genera *Hartmanella* or *Acanthamoeba*. The parasites enter the nervous system through the cribriform plate at the perforations for the olfactory nerves. An especially lethal form of this meningoencephalitis may develop with *Naegleria* spp. Other parasites, such as *S. mansoni*, may be acquired through swimming in contaminated freshwater, but it is unlikely that other parasites reach the nervous system through direct invasion across the cribriform plate. Schistosomiasis is acquired when the cercarial phase of the organism penetrates the swimmer's skin and finds its way into the blood.

147. The answer is e. (*Bradley, pp 1524–1525, 1590.*) The microglial nodules occurring with HIV are associated with syncytial cells in the brain and spinal cord, a cell type not typically seen with cytomegalovirus (CMV) encephalitis. Cytomegalovirus is a common CNS opportunistic agent in patients with AIDS. With HIV infection, the microglial nodules are distributed around blood vessels throughout the brain. With CMV, the nodules are more characteristically subpial and subependymal.

148. The answer is d. (*Victor, pp 768–770.*) B. burgdorferi is the agent responsible for Lyme disease. It is a spirochete usually transmitted to humans through tick bites. Multiple organ systems are attacked by the spirochete; the nervous system is especially susceptible. Erythema chronicum migrans is an expanding reddish discoloration of the skin that spreads away from the site of the bite as an expanding ring of erythema. It usually evolves over 3 to 4 weeks. This ring of erythema clears spontaneously within about 1 month and is usually associated with some headache and neck stiffness. Some patients with Lyme disease fail to exhibit the rash.

149. The answer is d. (*Victor, pp 793–795.*) The periodic discharges seen with herpes encephalitis typically occur over the temporal regions. Slow waves, rather than sharp waves, may be evident over the temporal lobes in many persons with severe disease. Seizures commonly occur early in the course of herpes encephalitis, so the EEG may be severely disturbed generally.

150. The answer is b. (*Victor, pp 768–770.*) If there is meningeal involvement, high-dose penicillin or ceftriaxone must be given intravenously for 10 to 14 days. Tetracycline qid for 30 days should be used for patients who are allergic to the intravenous treatments.

151. The answer is a. (*Victor, pp 752–756.*) There are many bases for abscess formation in the brain, but the most frequent causes are blood-borne infections from sources in the lung, heart, sinuses, and ears. Extension of infection from a chronic otitis or mastoiditis was much more common before the introduction of antibiotics. Facial or dental infections may spread to the brain through valveless veins draining about the muscles of mastication and communicating with the venous drainage of the brain.

152. The answer is d. *(Victor, pp 752–756.)* Brain abscesses usually start from a microscopic focus of infection at the junction of gray matter and white matter. As the infection develops, a cerebritis appears, and subsequently this focus of infection becomes necrotic and liquefies. Around the enlarging abscess there is usually a large area of edema.

153. The answer is a. *(Bradley, pp 1534–1535.)* No antiviral therapy affects the course of rabies. Immunization against rabies after exposure has occurred is essential, though even this may not substantially improve the outlook of this almost invariably fatal disease. The infected patient must receive intensive care, with precautions taken to prevent spread of the virus through contact with body fluids, such as saliva. Transmission of the virus through casual contact does not seem to occur, but it may be transmitted through corneal transplantation when the donor has been infected. Zidovudine (azidothymidine, AZT) is an antiretroviral drug useful in slowing the progression of HIV-1 infection. Ganciclovir has found increasing use in the management of cytomegalovirus (CMV) infection, especially when CMV involves the eye in a chorioretinitis. Amantadine was developed as an anti-influenzal agent, but it is used primarily to reduce the symptoms of Parkinson's disease. The reason for its antiparkinsonian action is unknown.

154. The answer is b. *(Bradley, p 1497.)* A gumma is a largely or entirely avascular granuloma. It rarely develops intracranially, but when it does, it may grow to several centimeters across. The lesion starts as an inflammatory process but becomes fibrosed as it evolves. The term *gumma* has traditionally been reserved for granuloma-like lesions caused by spirochetal infection.

155. The answer is e. *(Bradley, pp 1534–1535.)* Rabies is usually spread through the saliva of an infected animal. Introduction of saliva into a bite wound allows the virus to inoculate muscles or subcutaneous tissues. After introduction of the virus, the incubation period until fulminant infection appears extends from a few days to over 1 year, but usually ranges from 1 to 2 months. Bites of the head and face carry the greatest risk of causing fatal disease. Early after exposure, the patient will often complain of pain or paresthesias at the site of the animal bite. Animals transmitting the virus include dogs, bats, skunks, foxes, and raccoons. Dehydration as a complication of rabies is no longer likely because intravenous fluids can be given to completely replace what the hydrophobic patient cannot consume by mouth. Other complications of rabies include a paralytic form of the disease that progresses to quadriplegia (dumb rabies) in 20% of patients. With the classic form of the disease, the patient will also exhibit intermittent hyperactivity.

156. The answer is d. (*Victor, p 773.*) Patients with brain abscesses may exhibit focal signs, seizures, delirium, or less specific neurologic findings. These patients often have fever, but the CSF may not reflect the infectious basis of the fever until the abscess ruptures into the ventricles or subarachnoid space. Although *Aspergillus* is the most common cause of fungal abscesses, it is a relatively uncommon cause of fungal meningitis or meningoencephalitis. *Nocardia* is not classified as a fungus despite its resemblance to a fungus.

157. The answer is d. (*Bradley, p 1497.*) General paresis is a slowly evolving process that may require years to produce substantial disability. The early symptoms are a subtle dementia, characterized by memory loss and impaired reasoning, with later development of dysarthria, myoclonus, tremor, seizures, and upper motor neuron signs, leading to a bedridden state. Both the meninges and the parenchyma of the brain are involved by this chronic infection. The meninges are thickened and opaque, and a granular ependymitis characteristically develops. Degenerative changes occur throughout the cerebral parenchyma. Penicillin is the treatment of choice for this disease. The damage done to the brain is not mediated by autoimmune or adverse drug reaction mechanisms. This infection produces widespread injury to the brain rather than the restricted brainstem damage that typically occurs with infections that attack structures arising from the embryonic rhombencephalon. With a rhombencephalitis, the pons and medulla oblongata are the principal targets of disease.

158. The answer is b. (*Bradley, p 1592.*) Fungal abscesses develop with unusual frequency in patients with AIDS, but *T. gondii*, an obligate intracellular parasite, is considerably more common than fungi as the cause of abscess formation. The fungi that do produce abscesses in persons with AIDS are most often *Cryptococcus, Candida, Mucor,* and *Aspergillus.* Mycobacteria and atypical mycobacteria are also common causes of abscess formation in some populations.

159. The answer is e. *(Victor, p 796.)* Mumps, measles, and varicella zoster infection appear to be acquired primarily by way of the respiratory tract. The poliovirus is an enterovirus, which means it enters primarily through the gastrointestinal tract. Rabies is transmitted by animal bites and reaches the CNS by migration in neuronal processes, presumably as it is swept along by retrograde axoplasmic flow. This is believed to be an unusual method of viral spread to the CNS. Most viruses that do produce CNS disease are carried to the CNS in the bloodstream rather than along neuronal processes with infected axoplasm.

160. The answer is c. *(Victor, p 754.)* Three-fourths of patients with brain abscess have headache. This usually develops within a few weeks of the appearance of the abscess. Only one-third of patients present with seizures or focal neurologic deficits. Only one-fourth exhibit papilledema. Brain abscesses may produce remarkably few changes in the CSF until the abscess penetrates into the subarachnoid or intraventricular space. Abscesses that have not yet communicated with the CSF will usually produce only a moderate elevation in the CSF protein content. If the abscess is unsuspected and untreated, it will usually extend to the ventricles. With perforation into the ventricle, the abscess usually proves fatal. The treatment of choice for brain abscess is surgical resection.

161. The answer is a. *(Victor, pp 752–756.)* Both aerobic and anaerobic streptococcal bacteria occur in more than half of all brain abscesses. *Staphylococcus aureus* most often occurs in patients who have had penetrating head wounds or have undergone neurosurgical procedures. Enteric bacteria (e.g., *Escherichia coli, Proteus,* and *Pseudomonas*) account for twice as many abscesses as *S. aureus*.

162. The answer is e. *(Bradley, pp 1621–1622.)* This patient has a subacute to chronic progressive disease characterized by a combination of dementia, tremor, ataxia, and myoclonus. The EEG and MRI findings are typical of a spongiform encephalopathy. Multi-infarct dementia and subarachnoid hemorrhage would be expected to produce at least one very discrete event, and the imaging studies would be expected to show evidence of infarcts or other vascular abnormalities. Friedreich's disease may produce some dementia, but it is not a prominent part of the clinical deterioration. This patient is also much older than would be consistent with Friedreich's disease.

163. The answer is b. (*Bradley, pp 1483–1484.*) *L. monocytogenes* meningitis develops in renal transplant recipients, patients with chronic renal disease, immunosuppressed persons, and occasionally in otherwise unimpaired persons. It may also affect neonates. This type of meningitis is not usually seen in older children. It may on occasion lead to intracerebral abscess formation. Third-generation cephalosporins are inactive against *Listeria*, and ampicillin and gentamicin are recommended therapy. Neither ampicillin nor penicillin alone is bactericidal.

164. The answer is e. (*Bradley, pp 1617–1618.*) The most likely cause of spongiform encephalopathy in this middle-aged woman is Creutzfeldt-Jakob disease. This is classified as a prion disease and can be transmitted via infected nervous system tissue, including dura mater grafts, and occasionally via growth hormone preparations acquired from cadaver pituitary glands. A similar disease (kuru) occurs in Fore Islanders of New Guinea and is presumed to spread through the ritual handling or eating of human brain tissue. As of 1999, 113 cases due to growth hormone preparations had been reported, with incubation periods ranging from 5 to 30 years.

165. The answer is c. (*Bradley, pp 1594–1596.*) This patient probably had AIDS with PML as a complication of that disease. The inclusion bodies in the oligodendrocyte nuclei are JC virus, a papillomavirus. Primary infection with JC virus is universal and asymptomatic. Immunosuppression leads to reactivation of the virus. Diagnosis is typically made by MRI, which shows multiple focal well-defined white matter lesions that do not enhance or have mass effect. Cerebrospinal fluid PCR for JC virus is also available, obviating the need for brain biopsy in most cases. Treatment with cytarabine arabinoside has not been shown to be effective in clinical trials. Less than 10% of patients may experience spontaneous remission. PML may also develop with lymphomas, leukemias, or sarcoid, but the incidence of this disease in the U.S. population has expanded greatly since the dissemination of HIV in the population.

166. The answer is e. (*Victor, pp 1380–1387.*) The loss of strength associated with Guillain-Barré syndrome usually reaches a nadir within 2 weeks of the onset of symptoms. Sensation is usually preserved except for paresthesias in the feet or lower legs. Weakness is usually symmetric and often follows an ascending pattern of involvement. Tendon reflexes in the weak limbs are usually hypoactive or absent. Bladder and bowel control remain intact, but the patient usually exhibits some autonomic dysfunction, such as tachycardia and excessive sweating, which is rarely life-threatening. Eye muscles may be affected with Guillain-Barré syndrome, particularly in the condition called the Miller-Fisher variant. Before artificial ventilators were available, these patients often died from respiratory complications. The CSF with this disease typically reveals an elevated protein content with a relatively normal or only slightly abnormal white cell count and an invariably normal glucose content. This helps to distinguish it from poliomyelitis, a cause of paralysis that produces an alteration in both the protein and WBC content of the CSF consistent with a viral meningitis.

167. The answer is f. (*Victor, pp 766–767.*) Tabes dorsalis is caused by *Treponema pallidum,* the agent responsible for all types of neurosyphilis, but it is a disease entity distinct from general paresis, the form of neurosyphilis in which personality changes and dementia do occur. With tabes dorsalis, the patient develops a leptomeningitis. The posterior columns of the spinal cord and the dorsal root ganglia are hit especially hard by degenerative changes associated with this form of neurosyphilis. Tabes dorsalis is a form of neurosyphilis that usually becomes symptomatic decades after the initial treponemal infection. The gait ataxia and positive Romberg sign in this patient are manifestations of absent position sense. Bladder and bowel control may be profoundly disturbed, presumably on the basis of dorsal spinal root disease. The bladder is usually hypotonic (flaccid), and megacolon may develop. Patients with tabes dorsalis routinely exhibit abnormal (Argyll Robertson) pupils and optic atrophy. The glucose and glycohemoglobin should be checked to eliminate the more common cause of impaired position sense in the United States, diabetes mellitus. That this patient is from a part of the world that has relatively poor health care is relevant because this form of syphilis is rarely seen in persons who have spent most of their lives in countries with easy access to antibiotics.

168. The answer is b. (*Victor, pp 810–811.*) Subacute sclerosing panencephalitis usually develops in children and is rarely seen after the age of 18. Most affected children have had a bout of measles (rubeola) that occurred before they were 2 years old. SSPE may not appear for as long as 6 to 8 years after the episode of measles. Death usually occurs within 1 to 3 years after the onset of symptoms. SSPE produces a CSF pattern similar to that seen with multiple sclerosis, whose features include an increase in the gamma globulin fraction and the presence of oligoclonal bands. The measles virus appears to be directly responsible for this demyelinating disease, and the oligoclonal bands that appear in the CSF include a substantial proportion of measles-specific antibody. Eosinophilic inclusions are typically present in the cytoplasm and nuclei of neurons and glial cells.

169. The answer is h. (*Bradley, p 1504.*) Cat-scratch disease produces a regional adenitis, frequently involving epitrochlear nodes due to scratches on the patient's arm from an infected animal. The causative agent is *B. henselae* (rarely *Afipia felis*). In immunocompetent hosts, it may produce a self-limited aseptic meningitis. In HIV-infected individuals, it may produce a more virulent encephalitis associated with status epilepticus. Typically, these patients have disseminated disease, including distinctive skin lesions composed of neovascular proliferation (bacillary angiomatosis). On rare occasions, immunocompetent patients may have encephalitis as well. An MRI may show a characteristic increased signal intensity in the pulvinar, suggesting a tropism of the organism or immune response to this particular structure in the posterior thalamus.

170. The answer is g. (*Bradley, pp 1568–1573.*) Cysticercosis is produced by the larval form (cysticercus) of the pork tapeworm, *Taenia solium.* This is the most common neurological infection throughout the world, occurring most commonly in South America, Southeast Asia, and Africa. It is transmitted by fecal-oral contact; tapeworm eggs hatch in the human GI tract, invade the bowel mucosa, and migrate throughout the body, particularly into CNS, muscle, eye, and subcutaneous tissues. Cysticercal infection of muscles produces a nonspecific myositis. Brain involvement may lead to seizures. The lesions in the brain may calcify and often appear as multiple small cysts spread throughout the cerebrum.

Neoplasms

Questions

DIRECTIONS: Each item below contains a question followed by suggested responses. Select the **one best** response to each question.

171. A 65-year-old right-handed woman began having neurological problems about 1 week ago. She began experiencing nausea, vomiting, and numbness in the left hand and left foot. Today she had a generalized convulsion, and since then she has had a throbbing headache that is worse when she bends forward. On examination, the only deficits she has are loss of double simultaneous tactile stimulation and left lower facial droop when smiling. MRI reveals a lesion suggestive of a primary brain tumor. Which of the following is the most common source of primary brain tumors?

a. Glial cells
b. Neurons
c. Meningeal cells
d. Lymphocytes
e. Endothelial cells

172. A previously healthy 31-year-old man collapses in the kitchen of his home while sitting at the table talking. His wife witnessed a convulsion that lasted about 2 minutes. He seems to recover fully within an hour. The history taken in the ER reveals that he has been having new headaches in the early morning hours over the past few weeks. A brain MRI indicates that there is an enhancing right frontal lesion that is most likely a primary brain neoplasm. Which of the following is the most common type of primary brain tumor?

a. Meningioma
b. Astrocytoma
c. Lymphosarcoma
d. Oligodendroglioma
e. Medulloblastoma

173. Most brain tumors in children are which of the following?
a. Metastatic lesions from outside the central nervous system (CNS)
b. Oligodendrogliomas
c. Glioblastomas multiforme
d. Meningiomas
e. Infratentorial

174. The incidence of primary brain tumors in children—about 1 to 5 per 100,000 per year—is mainly accounted for by which of the following?
a. Meningiomas and neurofibromas
b. Astrocytomas and medulloblastomas
c. Melanomas and choriocarcinomas
d. Gliomas and adenomas
e. Colloid cysts of the third ventricle

175. A 72-year-old woman has a head CT performed because of headaches. It is significant for a left hemisphere mass with an overlying hyperostosis of the skull. She most likely has which of the following?
a. Meningioma
b. Pituitary adenoma
c. Astrocytoma
d. Schwannoma
e. Hemangioblastoma

176. A 9-year-old girl with papilledema and precocious puberty is most likely to have which of the following?
a. A pineal region tumor
b. An oligodendroglioma
c. A Kernohan class II astrocytoma
d. A brainstem glioma
e. An ependymoma

177. A 15-year-old boy has multiple angiomatoses of the retina and cysts of the kidney and pancreas. Which of the following brain tumors is most likely to develop in this child?

a. Glioblastoma multiforme
b. Meningioma
c. Hemangioblastoma
d. Ependymoma
e. Pinealoma

178. A 56-year-old right-handed woman who had breast cancer 1 year ago began having neurological problems about 1 week ago. She began experiencing nausea, vomiting, and numbness in the right hand and foot. Today she is experiencing crescendo pain in the left retroorbital area. Her headache is throbbing and positional, particularly when she tries to bend forward. The headache was intense in the morning, and at times it woke her up last night. On examination, the only deficits are loss of double simultaneous tactile stimulation and right lower facial droop when smiling. Which of the following is the most appropriate next action?

a. Administer intravenous prochlorperazine
b. Give the patient a prescription for zolmitriptan
c. Make a follow-up appointment for next month
d. Order an electroencephalogram to rule out seizures
e. Get a brain MRI

179. A 60-year-old woman presents to her internist with 2 months of new headaches and some difficulty walking. Further evaluation reveals multiple brain masses. Which of the following is the most common source of metastatic tumors to the brain in patients without a known primary tumor?

a. Breast
b. Lung
c. Kidney
d. Skin
e. Uterus

180. A 29 year-old woman with a history of malignant melanoma presents to her primary care doctor with a new type of headache. Examination is normal and a head CT is ordered. Multiple small brain hemorrhages are revealed by the scan. Metastatic lesions to the brain most often appear in which of the following locations?

a. At the gray-white junction
b. In the thalamus
c. In the posterior fossa
d. In the caudate
e. In the sella turcica

181. The shortest life expectancy with metastatic disease to the brain will be found in the patient with which of the following metastatic cancers?

a. Malignant melanoma
b. Breast cancer
c. Lung cancer
d. Renal cancer
e. Prostate cancer

182. A patient has an MRI performed and a colloid cyst of the third ventricle is identified. Which of the following is the most common complication of this lesion?

a. Bitemporal hemianopsia
b. Hydrocephalus
c. Gait ataxia
d. Optic atrophy
e. Oscillopsia

183. A 45-year-old right-handed man who has been HIV positive for the past 3 years has noticed some sort of visual change over the past 1 to 2 months. It is difficult for him to describe, but it is some sort of distortion of part of his right visual field. There is a 4-cm rim-enhancing lesion in the left occipital lobe that is revealed by MRI. Which of the following tumor types is common in the brain of patients with AIDS, but otherwise extremely rare?

a. Lymphocytic leukemia
b. Metastatic lymphoma
c. Primary lymphoma
d. Kaposi's sarcoma
e. Lymphosarcoma

184. A 37-year-old man presents with visual impairment. Examination reveals a bitemporal hemianopsia. Which of the following tumors is most likely responsible for this finding?

a. Optic glioma
b. Occipital astrocytoma
c. Brainstem glioma
d. Pituitary adenoma
e. Sphenoid wing meningioma

185. A 9-year-old girl presents with precocious puberty and episodes of uncontrollable laughter. Which of the following mass lesions might explain her symptoms?

a. Craniopharyngioma
b. Choroid plexus papilloma
c. Giant aneurysm
d. Metastatic carcinoma
e. Hypothalamic hamartoma

186. With an ependymoma of the posterior fossa, the patient is at risk of dying because of which of the following?

a. Transforaminal herniation
b. Emboli from the tumor
c. Vascular occlusion by the tumor
d. Hemorrhagic necrosis of the tumor
e. Status epilepticus

DIRECTIONS: Each group of questions below consists of lettered options followed by a set of numbered items. For each numbered item, select the **one** lettered option with which it is **most** closely associated. Each lettered option may be used once, more than once, or not at all.

Questions 187–191

Match each clinical scenario with the appropriate type of tumor.

a. Medulloblastoma
b. Oligodendroglioma
c. Optic glioma
d. Carcinomatous meningitis
e. Schwannoma
f. Choriocarcinoma
g. Metastatic carcinoma
h. Pineocytoma
i. Primary CNS lymphoma

187. A 30-year-old man with acquired immune deficiency syndrome (AIDS) develops headaches and left hemiparesis and is found to have a right frontal white matter homogeneously enhancing lesion.

188. A 4-year-old boy presents with ataxia, lethargy, and obstructive hydrocephalus.

189. A 16-year-old boy with café au lait spots and cutaneous nodules complains of decreased vision in his left eye.

190. A 55-year-old woman presents with mild unsteadiness, tinnitus, and hearing loss.

191. A 13-year-old girl has headaches and diplopia. On examination, she has impaired upward gaze, lid retraction, and convergence-retraction nystagmus. Her pupils react on convergence but not to light.

Questions 192–195

Match each clinical scenario with the most likely causative disorder.

a. Paraneoplastic cerebellar degeneration
b. Limbic encephalitis
c. Dorsal root ganglionopathy
d. Hypercalcemia
e. Cancer-associated retinopathy
f. Pseudotumor cerebri
g. Motor neuron disease
h. Guillain-Barré syndrome
i. Paraproteinemic neuropathy
j. Opsoclonus-myoclonus
k. Stiff-man syndrome
l. Lambert-Eaton myasthenic syndrome
m. Myasthenia gravis

192. A 67-year-old woman has a 2-month history of progressive gait disturbance. On exam, she has dysmetria of the limbs; a wide-based, unsteady gait; and hypermetric saccades. A hard, firm breast lump is discovered.

193. A 70-year-old man with a history of lung cancer develops nausea and vomiting and then becomes lethargic. On exam, he is lethargic but arousable, disoriented, and inattentive. He is weak proximally and has diminished reflexes.

194. A 57-year-old woman with a history of smoking has a 3-month history of hip and shoulder weakness. She also complains of xerostomia. There are no sensory symptoms, and she is cognitively intact. On exam, she is orthostatic. There is proximal muscle weakness, but she has increasing muscle strength with repetitive activity of her muscles. Eye movements are normal.

195. A 65-year-old woman develops pain and paresthesias in her feet. On examination, she has loss of reflexes, stocking distribution sensory loss, and mild distal weakness. Serum protein electrophoresis reveals a monoclonal gammopathy, and bone marrow biopsy reveals plasma cell dyscrasia.

Neoplasms

Answers

171. The answer is a. (*Bradley, p 1329.*) Between 2 and 5% of all tumors occurring in the general population are primary CNS tumors. In adults, the most common primary brain tumor is the astrocytoma. In children, brain tumors are more likely to arise in the posterior fossa. Even in childhood, glial cell tumors, such as the cerebellar astrocytoma and the optic glioma, are common.

172. The answer is b. (*Bradley, p 1329.*) The most common primary brain tumors are malignant astrocytomas. These are classified as grade 3 or 4. Grade 4 astrocytoma is more commonly called *glioblastoma multiforme.* It is malignant in the very conventional sense that it invades adjacent tissue. This type of glial tumor is usually seen in adults; men are more susceptible than women.

173. The answer is e. (*Bradley, p 1423.*) The posterior fossa is the usual location for brain tumors in children. Medulloblastomas, ependymomas, and cerebellar (or brainstem) gliomas account for most of the tumors that occur before puberty. Other common tumors developing intracranially in children include optic gliomas and metastatic leukemias.

174. The answer is b. (*Bradley, pp 1423–1424.*) Meningiomas may occur in childhood, but are more likely to appear and become symptomatic during adult life. Neurofibromas are not primary brain tumors, although schwannoma of the eighth cranial nerve is sometimes incorrectly referred to as an acoustic neurofibroma rather than an acoustic schwannoma. Colloid cysts of the third ventricle are not necessarily neoplastic, although most are assumed to have started as neoplasms rather than as developmental anomalies. Glioma is a broad category that includes the astrocytoma. Adenomas, such as pituitary adenomas, do develop in children, but much less commonly than either astrocytomas or medulloblastomas. Central nervous system tumors account for a large proportion of the tumors seen in childhood. In fact, they are second in frequency only to childhood leukemias and account for 15 to 20% of childhood tumors.

175. The answer is a. *(Bradley, p 1356.)* Hyperostosis is thickening of the bone and is much less commonly induced by tumors in or about the brain than is thinning of the bone. Thinning occurs especially with pituitary adenomas, which may cause erosions in the floor of the sella turcica as an early feature. Calcifications may develop in schwannomas or astrocytomas, but both of these tumor types will usually cause bony erosions where they impinge on the skull. Calcifications may develop in many primary or metastatic brain tumors, but calcification sufficient to be readily seen on a skull x-ray suggests an astrocytoma, meningioma, oligodendroglioma, or metastatic tumor. Calcification can be visualized on CT scan in about 17% of medulloblastomas. With meningiomas, hyperostosis may develop in the bone adjacent to the tumor even if there is no infiltration of the bone by the tumor.

176. The answer is a. *(Victor, pp 705–708.)* The pineal region is the source of an extraordinarily diverse group of tumor types, ranging from astrocytomas (derived from glial tissue) to chemodectomas (derived from sympathetic nervous tissue). Several different types of germ cell tumors arise from the tissues in this region, presumably from embryonal cell rests. In the United States, pineal tumors account for only 1% of intracranial tumors, but one-third of these pineal tumors are germ cell tumors, including germinomas and choriocarcinomas.

177. The answer is c. *(Bradley, pp 1894–1895.)* With von Hippel-Lindau syndrome, the patient may exhibit tumors in multiple organs. In the brain, hemangioblastomas are the tumors most likely to arise, and these tumors are usually limited to the cerebellum or brainstem. Hemangioblastomas are often multiple and become symptomatic by bleeding into themselves. The initial episode of bleeding may prove lethal.

178. The answer is e. *(Victor, pp 658–660, 684–686.)* The headache is typical of that caused by intracranial hypertension. Additionally, the patient has focal neurological symptoms and signs. This creates particular concern about a brain tumor or hemorrhage, and the patient should be evaluated as soon as possible. An appointment next month is too late. Intravenous prochlorperazine is a good treatment for status migrainosus; however, this history is atypical for such a diagnosis, and more serious problems should be ruled out first in the emergency room. Zolmitriptan is a treatment for migraines. This history is not typical for migraine, and zolmitriptan is also relatively contraindicated in patients with complex migraine. This history is very atypical for seizures, and an electroencephalogram is not likely to provide useful information in this case.

179. The answer is b. (*Bradley, p 1441.*) The breast, lung, kidney, skin, and uterus are all common sources of metastases to the brain. The incidences of metastases from the lung account for two-thirds of cases of brain metastasis presenting without a known primary. Skin lesions metastasizing to the brain include malignant melanomas.

180. The answer is a. (*Bradley, p 1442.*) Metastatic lesions are spread primarily by the vascular system. The gray-white junction (where the white matter and the gray matter meet) is the interface at which bloodborne cells are most likely to lodge and grow. No part of the brain is exempt from the spread of metastases, but the cerebral hemispheres and the cerebellum are especially vulnerable.

181. The answer is a. (*Victor, pp 697–699.*) The outlook with malignant melanoma, breast cancer, lung cancer, or renal cancer metastatic to the brain is poor and limited to a matter of months, but malignant melanoma is especially grim because it is highly likely to bleed after it metastisizes to the brain. Malignant melanoma and choriocarcinoma are likely to produce lethal intracranial hemorrhages, and the former may in fact first become apparent only after it has precipitated an intracranial hemorrhage. Prostate cancer does not typically metastasize to the brain.

182. The answer is b. (*Victor, pp 708–709.*) Colloid cysts may produce transient or persistent obstruction of the flow of CSF. Because this is an especially deep-seated lesion, it may be more practical to simply shunt the fluid from the lateral ventricles rather than attempt to excise the cyst. These cysts are usually lined with epithelial cells and may arise from a variety of sources, including low-grade neoplasms that involute early in their evolution.

183. The answer is c. (*Victor, pp 693–696.*) Kaposi's sarcoma is unusually common in patients with AIDS, but it is rarely metastatic to the brain. Metastatic lymphomas producing meningeal lymphomatosis are not especially rare in the general population, but primary lymphomas (i.e., lymphomas apparently arising in the CNS) were rare before the AIDS epidemic. The primary brain lymphoma usually presents as a solitary mass and can occur anywhere in the brain, but it does have a predilection for the periventricular structures.

184. The answer is d. *(Victor, p 714.)* With bitemporal hemianopsia, the visual fields in both eyes are impaired, but only the temporal quadrants of the field in each eye are affected. Pressure on the optic chiasm inferiorly by a tumor arising in or near the sella turcica will crush the fibers crossing in the chiasm from the medial aspects of the optic nerves. The most medial fibers in both optic nerves are contributed by the nasal aspects of the retina. The nasal or medial aspects of the retina receive light from the temporal or lateral aspects of the visual field.

185. The answer is e. *(Swaiman, pp 1058–1050. Victor, pp 594–595.)* Hypothalamic hamartomas are nonneoplastic malformations involving neurons and glia in the region of the hypothalamus. They may be discovered incidentally, either on imaging performed for other reasons or at autopsy, or they may cause symptoms referable to the hypothalamus. Most often, the latter involves neuroendocrine functions, causing precocious puberty or acromegaly due to overproduction of growth hormone–releasing hormone. Patients may also experience paroxysms of laughter, known as gelastic seizures. They may be cured surgically. Craniopharyngiomas are epithelial neoplasms arising in the sellar and third ventricular regions. They may cause hypopituitarism and visual field disturbances. Choroid plexus papillomas usually develop intraventricularly and do not extend down into the sella turcica. These tumors affect both children and adults, but they are rare. They are benign if they are surgically accessible and are extirpated early in their evolution. Giant aneurysms occur in many locations, but typically do not cause gelastic seizures or precocious puberty. Metastatic carcinoma generally occurs in older patients and would not be expected to cause these symptoms.

186. The answer is a. *(Bradley, p 1062.)* As a tumor of the posterior fossa enlarges, the contents of the posterior fossa will be compressed and ultimately forced upward or downward. If the herniation is upward, it is called *transtentorial* because it is across the tentorium cerebelli. If it is downward, it is called *transforaminal* because it is across the foramen magnum. Ependymomas are not especially vulnerable to hemorrhagic necrosis. Tumors in the posterior fossa generally do not produce seizures.

187. The answer is i. *(Bradley, p 1412.)* Patients with AIDS are at risk for numerous CNS infections, but have an increased frequency of only two tumor types: lymphoma and Kaposi's sarcoma. KS may metastasize to the CNS, but lymphoma is routinely primary to the CNS. This tumor may produce blindness through direct invasion of the optic nerve.

188. The answer is a. *(Swaiman, pp 1065–1067.)* Medulloblastomas are one of the most common CNS tumors of childhood. They typically develop in the cerebellum, causing ataxia. Astrocytomas may also occur in children infratentorially, primarily in the cerebellum and brainstem. In either location, hydrocephalus may develop because of obstruction at the level of the fourth ventricle. The astrocytoma that develops in the cerebellum is usually cystic. Medulloblastomas are invariably infratentorial, at least initially. They may extend supratentorially or become disseminated supratentorially through seeding of cells carried in the CSF. Ependymomas, another common tumor type in children, are derived from the lining of the ventricles and also carry the risk of hydrocephalus and seeding throughout the CNS.

189. The answer is c. *(Victor, p 719.)* The neurofibromatoses are a pair of hereditary neurocutaneous syndromes that result in a variety of congenital and later-occurring abnormalities and neoplasms affecting the skin, nervous system, and other organs. Neurofibromatosis (NF) type 1, also called peripheral NF, is characterized by café au lait spots, which are light to dark brown spots found on the skin; multiple cutaneous and subcutaneous tumors; bone cysts; sphenoid bone dysgenesis; precocious puberty; pheochromocytoma; syringomyelia; glial nodules; cortical dysgenesis; and macrocephaly. Optic nerve tumors are a particularly worrisome complication, and may produce blindness in children.

190. The answer is e. *(Victor, pp 709–712.)* Schwannomas usually develop on the vestibular division of cranial nerve VIII and are pathologically derived from Schwann cells rather than nerve tissue, and are therefore more appropriately called vestibular schwannomas than acoustic neuromas, the traditional name. Although this is not the division of the nerve that carries information from the cochlea, the cochlear division is crushed as the tumor expands. This type of tumor is especially likely with neurofibromatosis type 2, a hereditary disorder characterized by a variety of tumors in the skin and nervous system.

191. The answer is h. (*Victor, pp 705–708.*) Pineocytomas are histologically benign lesions affecting the region of the pineal gland. They arise from the parenchymal cells of the pineal gland. This patient's symptoms and signs constitute Parinaud syndrome, which may include loss of vertical gaze, loss of pupillary light reflex, lid retraction, and convergence-retraction nystagmus, in which the eyes appear to jerk back into the orbit on attempted upgaze. This syndrome occurs in lesions due to involvement of the dorsal midbrain in the region of the superior colliculus. Other tumors appearing in the pineal region that can produce a similar clinical picture include germ cell tumors (germinomas), teratomas, and gliomas. Malignant pineal tumors, or pineoblastomas, may also occur, and are similar histologically to medulloblastomas.

192. The answer is a. (*Victor, pp 724–725.*) Paraneoplastic cerebellar degeneration (PCD) is characterized by subacute and relentlessly progressive ataxia, dysarthria, and nystagmus. Myoclonus, opsoclonus (irregular jerking of the eyes in all directions), diplopia, vertigo, and hearing loss may also occur. Imaging may eventually reveal cerebellar atrophy, and pathology will disclose loss of Purkinje cells in the cerebellum as the primary abnormality. The most common associated tumor types are small cell carcinoma of the lung, ovarian carcinoma, and lymphoma, in that order. Approximately 50% of patients may harbor anti–Purkinje cell antibodies (called anti-Yo antibodies), and these are especially commonly found in women with breast cancer or other gynecologic malignancies. Interestingly, the symptoms of PCD often precede the symptoms of the underlying tumor itself, leading to speculation that the immune reaction that damages the nervous system may, in fact, be protective against the tumor.

193. The answer is d. (*Bradley, p 1690.*) Hypercalcemia may occur as a complication of cancer in up to 5% of patients. It may be a result of parathyroid-related peptide secreted by the tumor itself (usually a lung cancer) or of bone destruction by metastatic disease. The elevated serum calcium decreases membrane excitability, leading to the clinical syndrome of fatigability, lethargy, generalized weakness, and areflexia. In more severe cases, coma and even convulsions can occur. Symptoms usually do not occur until levels reach 14 mg/dL or higher.

194. The answer is l. (*Victor, pp 1547–1549.*) The Lambert-Eaton myasthenic syndrome (LEMS) shares some features with myasthenia gravis, notably proximal muscle weakness. It usually develops subacutely, however, and spares the bulbar musculature and eyes. There is also little response to anticholinesterase drugs. A characteristic feature is the increase in strength briefly after repeated muscle activation. Most cases are associated with an underlying oat cell carcinoma of the lung or other malignancy. In other cases, LEMS may be associated with other autoimmune illness. The underlying defect is the loss of function of the voltage-sensitive calcium channels in the presynaptic nerve terminal at the neuromuscular junction, due to cross-linking and aggregation by pathologic IgG autoantibodies. Various immune-modulating therapies, as well as 3,4-diaminopyridine, have been used with varying success. Removal of the underlying malignancy may also be curative.

195. The answer is i. (*Bradley, pp 1087, 2352.*) Polyneuropathy may occur in up to 15% of patients with multiple myeloma. This generally takes the form of a chronic distal symmetrical sensory or sensorimotor neuropathy. In some cases, the neuropathy progresses more aggressively, and the patient becomes confined to a wheelchair. Spinal fluid protein may be elevated, and the illness has the appearance of a chronic inflammatory demyelinating polyneuropathy. Up to 20% of patients referred for evaluation of polyneuropathy may have an underlying monoclonal paraproteinemia. In the absence of an obvious malignancy, this is called a monoclonal gammopathy of undetermined significance, but a hematologic malignancy may later turn up in as many as one-third of such patients.

Nutritional and Metabolic Disorders

Questions

DIRECTIONS: Each item below contains a question followed by suggested responses. Select the **one best** response to each question.

196. In Tay-Sachs disease, the enzymatic abnormality responsible for the neurologic deficits is deficiency of which of the following?
a. Hexosaminidase A
b. Glucocerebrosidase
c. Phosphofructokinase
d. Glucose phosphorylase
e. Sphingomyelinase

197. With β-glucosidase deficiency, the affected child is likely to exhibit abnormal accumulations of which of the following?
a. Glucosylceramide
b. G_{M2} ganglioside
c. Galactosyl sulfatides
d. Sphingomyelin
e. Trihexosylceramide

198. A 53-year-old left-handed man presents with asterixis, esophageal varices, splenomegaly, and abdominal ascites. He is likely to exhibit altered consciousness on the basis of which of the following?
a. Renal tubular acidosis
b. Impaired hepatic detoxification of portal blood
c. Splenomegaly-induced anemia
d. Copper intoxication
e. Vitamin B_{12} deficiency

199. A patient has had progressive, chronic liver failure for the past 5 years. At the time of death, he would be expected to exhibit changes in which type of brain cells?

a. Oligodendrocytes
b. Striatal neurons
c. Pigmented cells of the substantia nigra
d. Astrocytes
e. Inferior olivary neurons

200. A 42-year-old man presents to the emergency room with seizures, mental status change, and vision difficulties. An MRI reveals an abnormally high T2 signal in the posterior cerebral white matter. There is proteinuria, and blood pressure is 210/120. The cerebrospinal fluid (CSF) protein content of this patient is likely to be which of the following?

a. Abnormally low
b. Normal
c. Elevated, but less than 100 mg/dL
d. Elevated to between 500 and 1000 mg/dL
e. Greater than 2000 mg/dL

201. A 65-year-old man has had many years of deteriorating kidney function due to diabetes. At age 59, dialysis was begun because of electrolyte abnormalities. Which of the following is the most common neurologic complication of chronic renal failure?

a. Peripheral neuropathy
b. Delirium
c. Seizures
d. Dementia
e. Labile affect

202. A 70-year-old woman with end-stage renal disease tends to develop restless legs syndrome as she becomes uremic. This may be controlled with which of the following drugs?

a. Haloperidol
b. Clonazepam
c. Caffeine
d. Nifedipine
e. Rifampin

203. A 56-year-old woman has been on dialysis for the past 10 years due to chronic renal failure from cystic kidney disease. Which of the following is the most reliable treatment for the peripheral neuropathy associated with her condition?

a. Thiamine supplements
b. Clonazepam
c. Phenytoin
d. Minoxidil
e. Renal transplant

204. A 68-year-old man presents with acroparesthesia, sensory ataxia, memory loss, and impotence. On exam, there are upper motor neuron signs in all four extremities. He also has anemia and a sore tongue. Eventually, vitamin B_{12} deficiency is diagnosed. For vitamin B_{12} to be absorbed, it must bind to which of the following?

a. A cyanide atom and form cyanocobalamin
b. An intrinsic factor
c. The parietal cells of the stomach
d. The ileal mucosa
e. The jejunal mucosa

205. With vitamin B_{12} deficiency, which of the following accumulates in the blood?

a. Cysteine
b. Methylmalonic acid
c. Methionine
d. Succinic acid
e. Propionic acid

206. The patient with impaired vitamin B_{12} absorption is likely to develop a positive Romberg test because of damage to which of the following?

a. Cerebellar vermis
b. Cerebellar hemispheres
c. Spinal cord lateral columns
d. Basal ganglia
e. Spinal cord posterior columns

207. Which of the following types of visual field cuts is most often seen with vitamin B$_{12}$ deficiency?

a. Centrocecal scotoma
b. Homonymous hemianopsia
c. Bitemporal hemianopsia
d. Binasal hemianopsia
e. Hemianopsia with central sparing

208. A 42-year-old woman is being treated with methotrexate for Wegener's granulomatosis. She is at risk for megaloblastic anemia and peripheral neuropathy because methotrexate disturbs the metabolism of which of the following?

a. Cobalamin
b. Iron
c. Copper
d. Pyridoxine
e. Folate

209. A 37-year-old woman develops cholecystitis and requires cholecystectomy. Her family advises the physicians involved that she has a long history of alcoholism and benzodiazepine use, including diazepam (Valium), lorazepam (Ativan), and clonazepam (Klonopin). Approximately 7 days after the surgery, the patient becomes increasingly agitated, delusional, and suspicious. Routine investigations reveal no evidence of focal or systemic infection. Hepatic, renal, and hematologic parameters are largely normal. Within 24 h of these cognitive and affective changes, the patient has a generalized tonic-clonic seizure. Magnetic resonance imaging (MRI) and computed tomography (CT) studies of the brain are normal, and her CSF is unremarkable. In consideration of the abuse history provided by the family, medication orders prior to the surgery should have included which of the following?

a. Haloperidol
b. Chlorpromazine
c. Trihexyphenidyl
d. Prochlorperazine
e. Thiamine

210. A 55-year-old right-handed man is admitted to the medical service for pneumonia. The patient normally drinks 4 to 8 beers per day. In anticipation of the seizures, cognitive deterioration, and autonomic instability that might occur during withdrawal, which of the following is the most appropriate measure to take?

a. Consult a "detox center" to start planning the patients discharge
b. Provide intravenous alcohol supplements to blunt the alcohol withdrawal
c. Provide intramuscular or oral chlordiazepoxide several times daily at a dose dictated by the patient's level of agitation
d. Start phenytoin as a single dose nightly
e. Delay pneumonia treatment until the risk of neurologic problems abates

DIRECTIONS: Each group of questions below consists of lettered options followed by a set of numbered items. For each numbered item, select the **one** lettered option with which it is **most** closely associated. Each lettered option may be used once, more than once, or not at all.

Questions 211–217

For each clinical scenario, select the nutritional deficiency that is most likely responsible.

a. Deficiency amblyopia
b. Vitamin B_{12} deficiency
c. Pyridoxine (vitamin B_6) deficiency
d. α tocopherol (vitamin E) deficiency
e. Vitamin D deficiency
f. Thiamine (vitamin B_1) deficiency
g. Nicotinic acid deficiency
h. Kwashiorkor
i. Vitamin C deficiency

211. A 26-year-old man develops hemoptysis and dyspnea over the course of 3 months. His physician suspects tuberculosis and starts him on triple therapy with isoniazid (isonicotinic acid hydrazide), rifampin, and ethambutol. After 1 month of treatment, the patient's liver enzymes show slight elevations, but the treatment is continued. The hemoptysis stops by 2 months, but the patient complains of pins-and-needles sensations in his feet. Neurologic examination reveals hypoactive deep tendon reflexes in the legs and slightly impaired position sense. Strength is good in all limbs.

212. A 50-year-old woman is found wandering in the street and is brought to the emergency room by the police. She is disoriented to time, place, and person, but has no evidence of head trauma. She staggers when she tries to walk, but she has no detectable alcohol in her blood. Eye movements are abnormal with paresis of conjugate gaze, and horizontal nystagmus is apparent. Relatives are contacted, and they report that this woman has a long history of alcohol abuse.

213. A 46-year-old man complains of progressive visual problems. He notices problems with discriminating objects both up close and far away. His deficits have progressed over the course of 3 months. He has a 12-year history of pipe smoking, a 14-year history of daily aspirin use, and a 20-year history of alcohol intake. He usually drinks 4 oz of gin daily. Examination reveals enlargement of the physiologic blind spot to the point where it extends into central vision.

214. A 32-year-old South African woman develops irritability, sleeplessness, and fatigue. Her family believes that she is depressed, but neurologic assessment establishes prominent short- and long-term memory problems. She has anemia and an obvious dermatitis on her face. Her diet is strictly vegetarian and limited almost entirely to grains, such as corn.

215. A 61-year-old man develops progressive cramping of his legs and a pins-and-needles sensation in his feet over the course of 1 year. He consults a physician when he notices paresthesias in his hands and unsteadiness of his gait. His family reports that he has had some urinary incontinence, but was too embarrassed to report it. On examination, he has a spastic paraparesis with severe disturbance of position and vibration sense in his legs. Despite obvious spasticity in the legs, the deep tendon reflexes are absent at the knees and ankles. Peripheral blood smear reveals hypersegmented polymorphonuclear leukocytes.

216. A 4-year-old boy develops progressive gait ataxia and limb weakness over the course of 3 months. Neurologic assessment reveals diffusely absent deep tendon reflexes, proximal muscle weakness, ophthalmoparesis, and poor pain perception in the feet. Blood tests reveal elevated creatine phosphokinase (CK) levels and abnormally high serum bilirubin levels. Further investigations of hepatic function reveal that the child has a cholestatic hepatobiliary disorder, but there is no evidence of hepatic dysfunction sufficient to cause an encephalopathy.

217. A 9-month-old girl from famine-stricken Ethiopia exhibits profound apathy and indifference to her environment. She is afebrile and appears to have no significant infections at the time of her initial evaluation. Her hair is sparse, and slight edema is evident about her ankles. She is well below the fifth percentile for height in her age group. With handling she becomes irritable, but throughout her examination she exhibits little spontaneous movement. Her mother reports having seen transient tremors in the girl's hands a few weeks earlier, but these abated after a few days.

Questions 218–224

For each clinical scenario, select the most likely diagnosis.
a. Postictal state
b. Hypothyroidism
c. Uremic encephalopathy
d. Wernicke's encephalopathy
e. Herpes encephalitis
f. Progressive multifocal leukoencephalopathy (PML)
g. Meningeal carcinomatosis
h. Central nervous system (CNS) toxoplasmosis
i. Multiple sclerosis
j. Hepatic encephalopathy
k. Subacute combined systems disease
l. Meningococcal meningitis
m. Subacute sclerosing panencephalitis (SSPE)
n. AIDS encephalopathy
o. Pickwickian syndrome

218. A 23-year-old woman with a history of hemophilia notices progressive memory difficulty. She has required little hematologic support, but she did receive transfusion of factor VIII at least five times over the past 7 years. Neurologic examination reveals word-finding difficulty, poor recent and remote memory, gait ataxia, mild dysarthria, and a labile affect. Her right plantar response is extensor and her left brachioradialis reflex is hyperactive with transient clonus. An MRI of the brain is unrevealing.

219. A 35-year-old businessman has sleep attacks. He runs a chain of dry-cleaning stores, but does not usually work with the cleaning fluids. He reports falling asleep several times during the workday, even at business meetings and during interviews. He has developed the sleep attacks only after gaining over 100 lb. His weight at the time of the examination is 324 lb.

220. A 19-year-old man develops obvious personality changes over the course of 2 weeks. He becomes agitated with little provocation and abuses his wife both verbally and physically. His behavior is sufficiently atypical for it to prompt his relatives to seek psychiatric assistance for him. While being interviewed by a psychiatrist, he becomes unresponsive and develops generalized convulsions with opisthotonic posturing, tonic-clonic limb movements, and urinary incontinence. He is hospitalized for investigation of his seizure disorder. On initial examination, he is noted to have a low-grade fever and a mild left hemiparesis. His CSF opening pressure is 210 mmH$_2$O. His CSF cultures yield no growth, and his EEG reveals polyspike-and-wave discharges originating in the right temporal lobe. A CT of his brain reveals focal swelling of the right temporal lobe.

221. A previously healthy 25-year-old woman develops acute loss of vision in her left eye. She awakens with pain in the eye and reduction of her acuity to perception of light and dark. She delays seeing a physician for 1 week, during which time her acuity gradually improves sufficiently to allow her to read. On examination, the physician discovers she has slurred speech and poor rapid alternating movements with the left hand. Ocular dysmetria is evident in both eyes. Her tandem gait is grossly impaired. The physician obtains an EEG, which is normal.

222. A 17-year-old man has headache and photophobia on awakening. His physician discovers a low-grade fever and resistance to neck flexion. The physician advises the patient to take acetaminophen and remain in bed for the next 24 h. Within 12 h, the patient develops nausea and more intense headache. He seems disoriented and inappropriately lethargic. His family brings him to an emergency room. The emergency room physician notes a petechial rash on the legs and marked neck stiffness. CSF examination reveals a glucose content of 5 mg/dL, protein content of 87 mg/dL, and cell count of 112 leukocytes, with 70% polymorphonuclear cells.

223. A 56-year-old man is struck over the parietal area of the head during a robbery. He loses consciousness for 35 min but has no focal weakness or numbness on recovering consciousness. Within 2 days of the incident, his wife finds him unresponsive in bed early in the morning. She calls for an ambulance, but before it arrives her husband becomes more alert and asks for something to eat, saying he wants to have some supper before he goes to bed for the night. The ambulance attendant first on the scene notes that the patient is disoriented to place and time and has weakness of his right arm and leg.

224. A 35-year-old woman is found unconscious on the floor of her apartment. A bottle of cleaning fluid is found on a table near her. One of the contents indicated in the fluid is carbon tetrachloride. The ambulance crew notes that the patient is breathing independently, but her breath has a distinctly fetid odor unlike that associated with the cleaning fluid. Her limbs are flaccid, and she groans when she is moved. She responds to no inquiries and is poorly responsive to pain. A serum ammonia level obtained at the emergency room is 250 mg/dL, triple the normal level. EEG reveals triphasic waves, most prominently over the front of the head.

Nutritional and Metabolic Disorders

Answers

196. The answer is a. (*Swaiman, pp 442–444.*) Children with Tay-Sachs disease die prematurely and exhibit mental retardation, seizures, and blindness. This is a ganglioside storage disease that occurs more commonly in Ashkenazi Jews than in the general population. The early-onset form will produce macrocephaly and a cherry red spot in the fundus.

197. The answer is a. (*Swaiman, p 452.*) The disease responsible for the accumulation of glucosylceramide is Gaucher's disease. Gaucher's disease is inherited as an autosomal recessive trait and may be diagnosed by demonstrating deficient glucocerebrosidase in fibroblasts or leukocytes. The severity of disease varies from nonneuronopathic types to acute infantile neuronopathic disease. Gaucher's disease produces hepatosplenomegaly and may cause lethal CNS disease. It is one of a collection of storage diseases called sphingolipidoses, which include Niemann-Pick disease, Krabbe's disease, and Fabry's disease. Fabry's disease involves the accumulation of another ceramide, trihexosylceramide. All the sphingolipids are nothing more than lipids that contain a sphingosine moiety. Sphingosine is a class of long-chain compounds with hydroxyl groups on carbons 1 and 3 and an amino group on carbon 2. They form ceramides by joining with fatty acids across the subterminal amino group. G_{M2} ganglioside accumulates in Tay-Sachs disease, and galactosyl sulfatides accumulate in metachromatic leukodystrophy.

198. The answer is b. (*Bradley, pp 1674–1675.*) The clinical picture presented suggests hepatic failure. Copper poisoning may lead to hepatic failure, but the altered consciousness would be a consequence of the liver disease rather than the heavy metal poison itself. Similarly, vitamin B_{12} deficiency may lead to dementia, but it would not produce the signs of hepatic insufficiency exhibited by this patient. Encephalopathy that develops with chronic hepatic disease and portal hypertension is often called portal-systemic encephalopathy because of the importance of toxin-laden blood's bypassing the liver as portal hypertension develops. Precisely what toxins produce the encephalopathy is still debatable, but ammonia is probably the most important one. This type of encephalopathy will develop if flow through the liver is obstructed and the liver is otherwise normal. This is distinct from the terminal coma that may develop with acute hepatic necrosis.

199. The answer is d. *(Bradley, p 1680.)* Long-standing hepatic disease may produce a profound encephalopathy, but changes in the brain are notably sparse with portal-systemic encephalopathy. The most obvious change is an increase in Alzheimer's type II astrocytes. These astrocytes are relatively large cells. Rare patients show more dramatic changes, which include neuronal loss and focal necrosis. With chronic alcoholism and hepatic insufficiency, patients exhibit a loss of Purkinje cells in the cerebellum, but this is a consequence of alcohol toxicity or thiamine deficiency rather than of toxic injury from the hepatic dysfunction.

200. The answer is c. *(Victor p 904.)* The elevation with hypertensive encephalopathy is variable because intracranial hemorrhage may occur with the hypertensive crisis, but most patients will have moderate increases in CSF protein. Lowering of the blood pressure may reduce the protein elevation.

201. The answer is a. *(Bradley, pp 2378–2379.)* The type of peripheral neuropathy most commonly developing with chronic renal failure is a symmetric, distal, mixed sensorimotor neuropathy. The legs are generally affected first and most severely. Men are more commonly affected than women. Most of the peripheral neuropathies in patients with chronic renal failure involve axonal degeneration. The neuropathy usually improves with dialysis.

202. The answer is b. *(Bradley, p 2047.)* The restless legs syndrome (Ekbom syndrome) is characterized by a feeling of discomfort in the legs that is relieved by movement. The sensation is felt deep within the limb, and is variably described as a pulling, stretching, or cramping. Restless legs syndrome occurs primarily at night, shortly after the patient lies down. It differs from akathisia, which is a restlessness that occurs during the daytime. It may be associated with peripheral neuropathy and anemia and is seen in patients with chronic renal disease, diabetes mellitus, and many other medical conditions. Exercise before going to bed may alleviate much of the discomfort. Agents that may be effective in alleviating symptoms include clonazepam, gabapentin, L-dopa, and opiates. Neuroleptics, calcium channel blockers, and caffeine may worsen symptoms.

203. The answer is e. (*Bradley, pp 2378–2379.*) B vitamins are generally replaced when patients receive dialysis. Thiamine is water-soluble and so is easily lost during dialysis, but even replacing thiamine is not nearly as effective in retarding or reversing the neuropathy of chronic renal failure as is renal transplantation. There are presumed to be neurotoxins in the blood of patients with uremia that are not removed by routine dialysis.

204. The answer is b. (*Bradley, pp 1695–1697.*) Intrinsic factor is a glycoprotein that is secreted by the gastric parietal cells. In most people with vitamin B_{12} deficiency, the problem is inadequate production of intrinsic factor rather than inadequate vitamin B_{12} in the diet. Persons with pernicious anemia usually have an atrophic gastritis with inadequate intrinsic factor production as a consequence. This is presumed to be mediated by an autoimmune disorder.

205. The answer is b. (*Bradley, pp 1695–1697.*) Vitamin B_{12} (cobalamin) is an essential cofactor in the conversion of L-methylmalonyl-CoA to succinyl-CoA and of homocysteine to methionine. Without sufficient vitamin B_{12}, the conversion of propionic acid to succinic acid is blocked, and the intermediate compound, methylmalonic acid, accumulates in the blood. It is readily excreted and may help in the diagnosis of cobalamin deficiency when it is found in excess in the urine. Serum homocysteine levels, but not cysteine levels, may also be elevated because the conversion of homocysteine to methionine is disrupted if vitamin B_{12} is not available to expedite the methylation of homocysteine. Without this conversion of homocysteine to methionine, folate metabolism is disturbed, which probably interferes with DNA synthesis in red blood cell (RBC) precursor cells.

206. The answer is e. (*Bradley, pp 1695–1697.*) Both the lateral and posterior columns of the spinal cord are damaged with cobalamin deficiency, but a positive Romberg sign develops with impaired position sense, a sensory modality carried in the posterior columns of the cord. Because both sensory and motor functions are disturbed with cobalamin deficiency, the resulting condition is called *combined systems disease.* The microscopic changes in the posterior and lateral columns of the spinal cord in the patient with combined systems disease include demyelination, gliosis, and vacuolar degeneration. The regions of the spinal cord most severely damaged are the lower cervical and upper thoracic. The vacuolar changes observed arise in the myelin sheaths of very large nerve fibers. Although this starts as a predominantly demyelinating lesion, it evolves into axonal loss. Patients develop spasticity and weakness, as well as disturbed vibration and position sense. The clinical picture becomes more confused because a peripheral neuropathy may also develop with cobalamin deficiency. The peripheral neuropathy of the sort occurring with vitamin B_{12} deficiency would ordinarily produce hyporeflexia. The lateral column damage, which involves the corticospinal tracts, would ordinarily cause hyperreflexia. Because both peripheral nerves and corticospinal tracts are damaged with vitamin B_{12} deficiency, the effect on reflexes is difficult to predict and often changes over time. The patient will usually start with hyperreflexia and then develop either clonus or hyporeflexia.

207. The answer is a. *(Bradley, pp 1695–1697.)* The blind spot that normally occurs in each eye enlarges and extends temporally to involve central vision in patients with chronic vitamin B_{12} deficiency. This is similar to the blind spot that is associated with alcohol and tobacco excess, a problem called tobacco-alcohol amblyopia. Tobacco-alcohol amblyopia also seems to develop because of a vitamin B deficiency, but the deficiency is presumed to be of thiamine rather than of cobalamin.

208. The answer is e. *(Kasper, p 602.)* Methotrexate inhibits dihydrofolate reductase, thereby interfering with the metabolism of folate. As is the case with cobalamin deficiency, this results in a megaloblastic anemia. Defective DNA synthesis underlies the marrow disturbance that is seen with both folate and cobalamin deficiencies.

209. The answer is e. *(Victor, pp 1211–1212.)* This woman was at risk for Wernicke's encephalopathy. She should have received supplemental thiamine for at least 3 days, even though this would not have prevented the cognitive deterioration that she exhibited. There was no indication for using a neuroleptic (e.g., haloperidol, chlorpromazine, or prochlorperazine), even though her alcohol and benzodiazepine use placed her at risk for developing a withdrawal psychosis. The anticholinergic trihexyphenidyl would not be appropriate as either a neuroleptic or an antiepileptic.

210. The answer is c. *(Victor, pp 1262–1263.)* Chlordiazepoxide at relatively high doses of 25 to 100 mg, four to six times daily, will usually block the more malignant features of both alcohol and benzodiazepine withdrawal. This drug is itself a benzodiazepine, but once the patient has passed through the withdrawal period for the drugs he or she has been taking, the chlordiazepoxide can be systematically and uneventfully reduced. There are no apparent advantages to using an antiepileptic such as phenytoin.

211. The answer is c. *(Victor, p 1395.)* Any patient treated with isoniazid must receive supplemental pyridoxine. Isoniazid does not interfere with pyridoxine absorption, but it does interfere with its participation in metabolic pathways. Persistently low pyridoxine activity leads to the development of a peripheral neuropathy. This is most likely to be seen as an isolated deficiency in patients on antituberculous therapy.

212. The answer is f. *(Victor, pp 1206–1212.)* An apparently acute deterioration in cognitive function in an alcoholic may stem from any one of several causes. Bleeding from esophageal varices may have produced a profound anemia. Inapparent head trauma may have produced a subarachnoid hemorrhage or subdural hematomas. If the patient's problem is due to a nutritional deficiency, it is most likely thiamine deficiency associated with alcoholism. That this patient has no alcohol in her blood at the time of the deterioration is irrelevant. The triad of dementia, gait difficulty, and oculomotor paresis is characteristic of Wernicke's encephalopathy, the rapidly progressive and potentially lethal form of thiamine deficiency. Peripheral neuropathy commonly develops with thiamine deficiency, but it is not a component of the encephalopathy caused by thiamine deficiency.

213. The answer is a. *(Victor, pp 1215–1216.)* The vitamin deficiency specifically responsible for injury to the optic nerve in persons who chronically smoke tobacco and drink ethanol is still uncertain. It probably arises from combined deficits of vitamins B_1, B_{12}, and riboflavin. This condition is also known as nutritional optic neuropathy and as tobacco-alcohol amblyopia. There has been considerable speculation about its arising as a consequence of chronic cyanide poisoning from tobacco smoking combined with vitamin B_{12} deficiency associated with alcoholism, but this theory has little support.

214. The answer is g. (*Victor, p 1217.*) Persons with limited diet devoid of animal fats and rich in corn are at risk for pellagra, a nutritional deficiency of nicotinic acid or its precursor, tryptophan. This disease typically affects the skin, digestive tract, central nervous system, and hematopoietic system. People with diets limited to corn (maize) are especially vulnerable because of the low levels of tryptophan and niacin in this grain.

215. The answer is b. (*Victor, pp 1218–1223.*) The slow evolution of gait difficulty, bladder dysfunction, paresthesias, hyporeflexia, impaired position and vibration sense, and anemia suggests combined systems disease, the neurologic equivalent of pernicious anemia. Persons with this disease may have a diet rich in vitamin B_{12}, but they will develop deficiency if they lack intrinsic factor in the stomach. Patients usually acquire a megaloblastic anemia associated with the spastic paraparesis. Finding hypersegmented polymorphonuclear cells on the peripheral blood smear helps establish the diagnosis.

216. The answer is d. (*Victor, p 1224.*) Vitamin E deficiency that causes neurologic disease is rare, but when it does develop it is usually during early childhood. The most common syndrome involves spinocerebellar degeneration, polyneuropathy, and pigmentary retinopathy. Clarke's columns, the spinocerebellar tracts, the posterior columns, the nuclei of Goll and Burdach, and sensory roots are especially likely to exhibit degeneration in persons with vitamin E deficiency. The most obvious symptom of the deficiency is likely to be ataxia.

217. The answer is h. (*Victor, pp 1227–1228.*) Protein deficiency states, such as those occurring with kwashiorkor, produce a wide range of neurologic signs and symptoms. Although the CNS is somewhat sheltered from the ravages of malnutrition, severe protein-calorie deficiencies during childhood development may leave the child neurologically impaired for life. Even when dietary supplements have been introduced to correct the chronic deficiency, the children are likely to exhibit little improvement in mobility or alertness for weeks or months.

218. The answer is n. *(Bradley, pp 1607–1609.)* This woman is at relatively high risk for AIDS encephalopathy because she has required transfusion of clotting factors that have until recently been available only from pooled samples of blood products. The neurologic deficits that she exhibits are not specific for HIV-1–associated subacute encephalomyelitis (AIDS encephalitis) and are quite compatible with multiple sclerosis (MS). That her MRI does not reveal plaques of demyelination scattered throughout the brain makes the diagnosis of MS improbable. To establish the diagnosis of AIDS encephalopathy, HIV-1 antibodies should be sought and the helper/suppressor (CD4/CD8) T lymphocyte ratio should be checked. Patients with symptomatic AIDS usually have a CD4/CD8 T lymphocyte ratio of less than 0.5.

219. The answer is o. *(Victor, p 421.)* Obesity associated with hypersomnia qualifies as pickwickian syndrome if the patient exhibits other characteristic features, such as sleep apnea. The patient with this syndrome is likely to have hypoxemia and pulmonary hypertension. Smoking increases the risk of developing the syndrome. Sleep attacks usually abate with cessation of smoking and weight loss.

220. The answer is e. *(Bradley, pp 1516–1518.)* With herpes encephalitis in the person who is not immunodeficient, the first clinical signs of disease are likely to be psychiatric. Depression, irritability, and labile affect are especially common. The organic basis for the encephalopathy usually becomes self-evident when the affected person has a seizure. Because the temporal lobe is especially involved by herpes encephalitis, the initial seizure is likely to be complex partial, but seizures often become more generalized. EEG will usually reveal the focal character of the cerebral damage. Intracranial pressure is usually increased with a fulminant infection. Temporal lobe swelling may be severe enough to produce lethal herniation.

221. The answer is i. *(Bradley, pp 1642–1645.)* Optic neuritis is often the first symptom that motivates the patient with multiple sclerosis to consult a physician. Clumsiness, stumbling, and other symptoms of ataxia are usually dismissed as inconsequential by the patient. Even those with profoundly slow and slurred speech are often unaware of their dysarthria. When the patient finally does consult a physician, multiple neurologic abnormalities are usually evident. This patient would be expected to have a positive swinging flashlight test (Marcus Gunn pupil) and evidence of widespread demyelination on MRI of the head.

222. The answer is l. *(Victor, pp 737, 739.)* With acute bacterial meningitis, the time between the first symptoms and death may be only days. A petechial rash developing over the lower parts of the body in the setting of fever, headache, nuchal rigidity, photophobia, and stupor must be considered presumptive evidence of a meningococcal meningitis. Rapid diagnosis and treatment is essential if the patient is to survive. The spinal fluid typically reveals a low glucose content, high protein content, and leukocytosis with a large number of polymorphonuclear cells. Treatment with intravenous penicillin G, 12 million to 15 million U daily (divided into four to six doses) early in the course of illness may decide whether the patient survives more than a few hours or days.

223. The answer is a. *(Bradley, p 17.)* After significant head trauma, the victim is at considerable risk for a seizure. A patient's seizure threshold is lowest when he or she is asleep or sleep-deprived. If the posttraumatic seizure occurs during sleep, it may go unnoticed. The patient's improving cognition suggests a postictal state. His hemiparesis is probably a Todd's paralysis, but any patient with posttraumatic seizures and focal weakness must be investigated for an acute or chronic subdural hematoma.

224. The answer is j. *(Victor, pp 1184–1188.)* Carbon tetrachloride is a potent hepatic toxin. This woman may have attempted to commit suicide by drinking cleaning fluid. As hepatic damage progressed, she developed fetor hepaticus, a distinctive smell to her breath that reflects a profound metabolic disturbance. The serum ammonia level rose as liver function declined. The triphasic waves typically seen in hepatic encephalopathy may occur with uremia and other causes of metabolic encephalopathy.

Dementia and Cognitive Disorders

Questions

DIRECTIONS: Each item below contains a question followed by suggested responses. Select the **one best** response to each question.

225. A 75-year-old woman with suspected normal-pressure hydrocephalus undergoes lumbar puncture. Forty milliliters of fluid are removed. Three hours later, she is able to walk unassisted and turns well. Spinal fluid would be expected to show which of the following?

a. No abnormalities
b. Elevated protein
c. Low protein
d. Atypical lymphocytes
e. Low glucose

226. A physician believes that her patient has Alzheimer's disease. Which of the following is most characteristic of the brain in patients with Alzheimer's disease?

a. Neuronal loss in the cerebral cortex
b. Demyelination in the cerebral cortex
c. Posterior column degeneration
d. Neuronal loss in the cerebellar cortex
e. Pigmentary degeneration in the hippocampus

227. An 80-year-old man has had a gradual memory decline over the past 10 years. A reversible cause of dementia cannot be found, and PET scan supports the diagnosis of Alzheimer's disease. In the dementia associated with Alzheimer's disease, the EEG will usually show which of the following?
a. Spike-and-wave discharges
b. Periodic frontal lobe discharges
c. Focal slowing
d. Generalized background slowing
e. An isoelectric record

228. A 55-year-old man has a steep decline in his cognitive abilities over a 3-month period. Initial testing is nondiagnostic. He continues to progress and develops myoclonus and a left hemiparesis. Eventually, he dies of an aspiration about 8 months after the onset of symptoms. In the diseases that cause dementia, myoclonus is usually most evident in which of the following?
a. Alzheimer's disease
b. Creutzfeldt-Jakob disease
c. Parkinson's disease
d. Huntington's disease
e. Pick's disease

229. A 29-year-old mentally retarded woman living in an institution has had a subacute to chronic decline in memory. Testing for reversible causes of dementia is nondiagnostic. The brain of the adult with trisomy 21 (Down syndrome) exhibits many of the histopathologic features of which of the following?
a. Tay-Sachs disease
b. Friedreich's disease
c. Pick's disease
d. Parkinson's disease
e. Alzheimer's disease

230. An 80-year-old man has a history of 2 years of progressive gait disturbance and incontinence, which had been attributed to old age and prostatism. Within the past 3 months, he has been forgetful, confused, and withdrawn. His gait is short-stepped, and he turns very slowly, almost toppling over. He has a history of head trauma from 30 years ago. His CT scan is shown below. Which of the following is the most likely diagnosis?

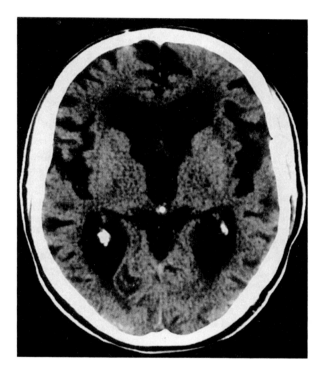

a. Alzheimer's disease
b. Creutzfeldt-Jakob disease
c. Progressive multifocal leukoencephalopathy (PML)
d. Normal-pressure hydrocephalus
e. Chiari malformation

231. An 82-year-old man has 6 months of worsening memory loss. His family is concerned, and he is taken to a physician. Following an extensive evaluation and neuropsychological testing, he is diagnosed with dementia. Which of the following is the most common cause of dementia in the general population?

a. Epilepsy
b. Vascular disease
c. Alzheimer's disease
d. Parkinson's disease
e. Head trauma

232. A patient undergoes ventriculoperitoneal shunt placement for hydrocephalus. He is discharged 2 days later, his gait and cognition much improved. The following morning, his wife finds him lying in bed, very confused and complaining of a headache. He is unable to walk. The surgeon who performed the procedure is concerned that these new symptoms are due to which of the following?

a. Chemical meningitis
b. Subdural hematoma
c. Epidural hematoma
d. Seizures
e. Bacterial ventriculitis

233. A 67-year-old man has a history of progressive memory loss for 2 years. His examination is otherwise normal. A diagnosis of Alzheimer's disease is made. Which of the following medications may result in some cognitive improvement?

a. Donepezil
b. L-dopa
c. Risperidone
d. Prednisone
e. Vitamin B_{12}

234. Language testing is most likely to uncover which of the following deficits in a patient with Alzheimer's disease?

a. No abnormalities
b. Mutism
c. Conduction aphasia
d. Transcortical sensory aphasia
e. Transcortical global aphasia

DIRECTIONS: Each group of questions below consists of lettered options followed by a set of numbered items. For each numbered item, select the **one** lettered option with which it is **most** closely associated. Each lettered option may be used once, more than once, or not at all.

Questions 235–240

For each clinical scenario, choose the most likely diagnosis.

a. Transient global amnesia
b. Normal-pressure hydrocephalus
c. Alzheimer's disease
d. Parkinson's disease
e. Creutzfeldt-Jakob disease
f. Vitamin B_{12} deficiency
g. Hypothyroidism
h. Huntington's disease
i. Rett syndrome
j. Multi-infarct dementia
k. General paresis
l. Temporal lobe epilepsy

235. A 73-year-old man steps out of the shower on a Saturday evening and is unable to remember that he and his wife have tickets to a play. He asks her repeatedly, "Where are we going?" He appears bewildered, but is alert, knows his own name, speaks fluently, and has no motor deficits. He has no history of memory disturbance, and after 8 h returns to normal.

236. A 50-year-old woman began having double vision and blurry vision 3 months ago and has since had diminishing interaction with her family, a paucity of thought and expression, and unsteadiness of gait. Her whole body appears to jump in the presence of a loud noise. An MRI scan and routine CSF examination are unremarkable.

237. A 2-year-old girl developed normally until the past year. She has since become unable to speak or otherwise communicate with her parents, sits in a chair, and makes nearly continuous wringing movements with her hands. She also has episodes of breath holding alternating with hyperventilation.

238. A 17-year-old girl develops mild dementia, tremor, and rigidity. Her father died in his fourth decade of life of a progressive dementing illness associated with jerking (choreiform) limb movements. On exposure to L-dopa, she becomes acutely agitated and has jerking limb movements.

239. A 62-year-old man has had 2 years of progressive memory loss and inappropriate behavior. He has been delusional. More recently, he has developed tremors, myoclonus, dysarthria, and unsteadiness of gait. The CSF shows a lymphocytic pleocytosis, protein of 150, and positive VDRL.

240. A 44-year-old woman from Africa presents with inattentiveness, poor concentration, and lethargy. She has paranoid delusions. There is mild proximal weakness and ataxia. On general exam, she has edema, coarse and pale skin, and macroglossia. On reflex examination, she has delayed relaxation of the ankle reflexes.

Questions 241–243

For each patient, select the likely organism that caused the disease.

a. HTLV-I
b. *Tropheryma whippelii*
c. *Treponema pallidum*
d. JC virus
e. Prion protein
f. Cytomegalovirus (CMV)
g. Herpes simplex virus
h. *Taenia solium*

241. A 54-year-old woman presents with 6 months of progressive memory loss. She has limited vertical eye movements, and on examination she has rhythmic, synchronous grimacing and eye closure movements (oculomasticatory myorhythmia). Jejunal biopsy reveals PAS-positive cells.

242. A 35-year-old intravenous drug abuser presents with inability to control his left hand. He reports that at times he will button his shirt with his right hand, only to find that his left hand is unbuttoning the shirt against his control. He has a history of thrush. He is alert and oriented. MRI shows an increased T2 signal affecting the subcortical white matter of the right parietal lobe without enhancement.

243. A previously healthy 24-year-old man presents with 3 days of headaches and fever, followed by hallucinations, speech disturbance, and lethargy. He has a mild right hemiparesis. Spinal fluid is bloody, and MRI shows abnormal signal, with enhancement, in the left anterior temporal lobe.

Dementia and Cognitive Disorders

Answers

225. The answer is a. (*Bradley, pp 1760–1762.*) The CSF in patients with NPH is typically normal. Abnormalities in protein or cellularity should suggest an alternative diagnosis. The pressure of the CSF is also usually normal, although studies using long-term pressure monitoring in these patients have shown that they have periods of pressure elevation, often at night.

226. The answer is a. (*Bradley, pp 1911–1913.*) The most prominent characteristics of Alzheimer's disease are neuronal loss, fibrillary tangles, loss of synapses, and amyloid (or neuritic) plaque formation. These histopathologic features are evident throughout the cerebral cortex, but the neurofibrillary tangles and neuronal loss are most prominent in the hippocampus and adjacent structures of the temporal lobe. The tangles and loss of synapses are most closely linked to the development of dementia. The cell loss may be so substantial that the patient develops marked compensatory enlargement of the ventricles, a condition called *hydrocephalus ex vacuo*.

227. The answer is d. (*Bradley, p 477.*) The background posterior dominant rhythm on the normal adult EEG is α activity at 8 to 12 Hz. With Alzheimer's disease, the frequency of this rhythm may slow, and the amount of time in which this rhythm is evident when the patient is lying relaxed with eyes closed may drop substantially. Periodic discharges in the form of sharp waves or spikes may develop during Creutzfeldt-Jakob disease. EEG is otherwise not especially helpful in distinguishing between the common causes of dementia.

228. The answer is b. (*Bradley, p 1941.*) Creutzfeldt-Jakob disease is a spongiform encephalopathy that produces dementia over the course of months. It is caused by the accumulation within the brain of an abnormal form of a normal protein that resists degradation by proteinases (a proteinase-resistant protein, prion protein, or PrP). Myoclonic jerks—

abrupt involuntary muscle contractions that may produce brief limb or facial movements—usually appear at some time in the course of this disease. These are often stimulus-sensitive, such that loud noises may provoke them. Similar movements may develop with Huntington's disease, but these patients usually develop more constant and fluid limb movements, called *chorea*.

229. The answer is e. *(Bradley, p 1915.)* Up to 90% or more of patients with trisomy 21 who die after age 30 have Alzheimer's-type changes in the brain. The histopathologic features of Alzheimer's disease may be evident in the person with Down syndrome at any age. That a hereditary form of Alzheimer's disease was found linked to chromosome 21 raised hopes that a single mutation was the cause of the problem, but this was subsequently negated by the finding of hereditary forms of Alzheimer's linked to chromosome 19 and sporadic Alzheimer's associated with defects on neither of these chromosomes. Aside from persons with Down syndrome, Alzheimer's disease only rarely develops in relatively young people.

230. The answer is d. *(Bradley, pp 1760–1762.)* Normal-pressure hydrocephalus (NPH) is a chronic, communicating form of hydrocephalus affecting elderly adults. The cause is unknown, but it may relate to prior episodes of trauma, infection, or subarachnoid hemorrhage. The clinical picture typically includes a triad of gait disturbance, dementia, and incontinence. The gait disorder, which may be difficult to distinguish from that of Parkinson's disease, has been labeled an apraxic gait, as patients often have difficulty even lifting their feet off the floor, though they have no weakness and may perform motor tasks well with the legs when seated. CT or MRI in these patients usually shows enlargement of the temporal and frontal horns of the lateral ventricles out of proportion to the degree of cortical atrophy. There may also be a squaring off or blunted appearance of the frontal horns, and increased signal on T2-weighted images may be seen in the periventricular regions, consistent with the presence of fluid related to transependymal flow of CSF.

231. The answer is c. *(Bradley, pp 1905–1906.)* Alzheimer's disease accounts for as much as 50% of the dementia in the general population confirmed at autopsy; Parkinson's disease accounts for only about 1%. Only 80 years ago, neurosyphilis was the most common cause of dementia, but the introduction of penicillin reduced—though it did not eliminate—this spirochetal disease as a cause of dementia. As the population ages, the incidence and prevalence of Alzheimer's disease are increasing. The dementia caused by Alzheimer's disease is progressive over the course of years. Language disturbances may appear even before memory problems.

232. The answer is b. *(Bradley, pp 1761–1762.)* Up to 28% of patients who undergo ventriculoperitoneal shunting for NPH may suffer major complications, including subdural hematoma. Subdural hematoma occurs because the reduction in intracranial pressure brought on by the reduction in CSF volume may cause the brain to pull away from the covering meninges, stretching and potentially rupturing the bridging veins.

233. The answer is a. *(Bradley, pp 1915–1917.)* Several modest advances in the treatment of Alzheimer's disease have occurred recently. Recognition of the fact that there is a cholinergic deficit in the brains of patients with Alzheimer's disease has led to the development of acetylcholinesterase inhibitors designed to augment the cholinergic neurotransmitter system. Two different agents that have been used for several years in the United States are tacrine, which can cause hepatic dysfunction, and donepezil, which is better tolerated. More recently, other cholinergic agonists and one drug with a different mechanism of action (memantine) have become available. The effects are modest and act to slow cognitive decline as assessed by scales of cognitive function. There is still no cure for Alzheimer's disease.

234. The answer is d. *(Victor, p 1110.)* The major clinical features of Alzheimer's disease are memory impairment, aphasia, apraxia, and neuropsychiatric impairment, including mood disturbances, delusions and hallucinations, personality changes, and behavior disturbances. The language disturbance may take the form of decreased fluency, dysnomia, and transcortical sensory aphasia, which refers to a reduction in the ability to understand complex linguistic structures. Repetition of verbal material is intact.

235. The answer is a. *(Bradley, p 71.)* Transient global amnesia (TGA) refers to an episode of complete and reversible anterograde and retrograde memory loss lasting up to 24 h. Patients have a persistent loss of memory for the time of the attack. During the episode, patients often appear bewildered and ask repeated questions. They retain personal identity (unlike characters suffering from transient amnesia in television shows) and can perform complex cognitive and motor tasks. Transient global amnesia usually affects middle-aged or older men and often occurs in the setting of an emotional or other stressor, such as physical or sexual exertion. Although it shares features of TIA, it is not associated with an increased risk of stroke. Nonetheless, a vascular evaluation is often appropriate, particularly in atypical or repeated cases and in the presence of risk factors for stroke. Most patients experience only a single episode. Some have stressed TGA's similarity to migraine and hypothesized that it is related to migrainous ischemia of the medial temporal lobe structures.

236. The answer is e. *(Bradley, pp 1941–1942.)* The neurological symptoms occurring early in the course of Creutzfeldt-Jakob disease are often cerebellar or visual. Patients may have ataxia, clumsiness, or dysarthria, as well as diplopia, distorted vision, blurred vision, field defects, changes in color perception, and visual agnosia. Ultimately, cortical blindness may occur. The diagnosis may be supported by the finding of periodic sharp waves at a 1- to 2-Hz frequency on EEG and the finding of elevated protein 14-3-3 in CSF. The typical EEG pattern is found in up to 80% of patients at some point during the course of the illness. An MRI may show a pattern of increased T2 signal in the basal ganglia or other gray matter in many, but not all, cases.

237. The answer is i. *(Swaiman, pp 612, 836–839.)* Rett syndrome is a presumed X-linked genetic disorder that affects only girls; the homozygous version is thought to be fatal in male offspring. Usually the prenatal, perinatal, and early childhood development appear normal or nearly so, and then the girl undergoes rapid regression in cognitive status in early childhood, generally during the second year of life. There is loss of previously acquired language skills and effective eye contact, as well as purposeful hand movement. Stereotypic hand movements develop, usually taking the form of hand wringing, but also include tapping, patting, and at times hand-mouth movements. Seizures may also occur. Etiology is unknown, and there is no treatment.

238. The answer is h. *(Bradley, pp 2148–2150.)* Dementia is a prominent feature of Huntington's disease. Apathy and depression occur commonly, and a schizophreniform illness may be the presenting manifestation at times. The dementia itself is subcortical, characterized by impairment in executive function and concentration, without the classic cortical features of Alzheimer's disease, such as aphasia, apraxia, and amnesia.

239. The answer is k. *(Victor, pp 765–766.)* General paresis is one of the manifestations of neurosyphilis. It is a chronic, often insidious meningoencephalitis that may be delayed up to 20 years after the original spirochetal infection. Clinically, it manifests as dementia, delusions, dysarthria, tremor, myoclonus, seizures, spasticity, and Argyll Robertson pupils. Diagnosis is based on the findings of a monocytic pleocytosis and positive serological tests for syphilis. When caught early and treated with penicillin, the prognosis for independence may be good in up to 40% of cases. Neurosyphilis may be asymptomatic. Its other symptomatic forms include meningitis, meningovascular syphilis causing infarcts, optic atrophy, tabes dorsalis (characterized by ataxia, urinary incontinence, and lightning pains due to degeneration of the posterior spinal roots), and other forms of spinal syphilis.

240. The answer is g. *(Bradley, p 1947.)* Hypothyroidism in adults may present with headache, dementia, psychosis, and decreased consciousness. Neuromuscular findings are also common, and they include a myopathic weakness and a delay in the relaxation phase of reflexes (the hung-up reflex). Percussion of muscles may also cause a mounding of the muscle, called *myoedema*. Cerebellar ataxia may also occur. In severe cases, myxedema coma may occur, characterized by hypothermia, hypotension, and respiratory and metabolic disturbances. This requires emergent replacement of thyroid hormone.

241. The answer is b. *(Bradley, p 1940.)* Whipple's disease is a rare multisystem disorder caused by *T. whippelii*. Gastrointestinal complaints, such as steatorrhea, abdominal pain, and weight loss, reflect bowel infection. Central nervous system infection, which may occur in the absence of GI disease, may produce seizures, myoclonus, ataxia, supranuclear gaze disturbances, hypothalamic dysfunction, and dementia. Oculomasticatory myorhythmia (pendular convergence movements of the eyes in association with contractions of the masticatory muscles) may occur and is considered pathognomonic. At times, other muscles of the body may be involved.

Diagnosis can be made by biopsy of the jejunum, though sometimes brain biopsy may be required and may show periodic acid–Schiff (PAS)-positive cells. Treatment with antibiotics may be curative, and, for this reason, the diagnosis is important to remember in unusual cases of dementia with movement disorders.

242. The answer is d. *(Bradley, p 1939.)* Progressive multifocal leukoencephalopathy is a progressive leukoencephalopathy seen in immunocompromised patients, most notably those with AIDS. It is caused by a papovavirus, usually the JC virus, but also SV-40 virus. The disease affects subcortical white matter, particularly in the occipital or parietal regions, leading to visual complaints or phenomena such as the alien hand syndrome, as in this patient. Cerebrospinal fluid is usually normal, and the lesions do not enhance on imaging studies. There are usually several foci of abnormality seen on MRI, which can be used reliably to make the diagnosis. In some cases, PCR detection of JC virus in the CSF can be used to make the diagnosis.

243. The answer is g. *(Bradley, p 1939.)* Herpes simplex virus (HSV) encephalitis is the most common form of sporadic encephalitis in the United States. Mortality approaches 70% without treatment, making early diagnosis crucial. Patients may present with acute onset of seizures or with a subacute course characterized by deficits referable to temporal lobe structures, such as amnesia, aphasia, or psychosis. Motor deficits also often occur. Headaches and fever are usually present. Eventually, declining level of consciousness and even coma may occur, and patients are at risk of uncal herniation from massive swelling of the temporal lobes. Electroencephalography, MRI, and CSF analysis help to confirm the diagnosis. Only in rare cases is biopsy needed. Mortality may be reduced to 20% with acyclovir.

Movement Disorders

Questions

DIRECTIONS: Each item below contains a question followed by suggested responses. Select the **one best** response to each question.

244. A 19-year-old pregnant patient gives a history of the recent onset of an involuntary movement disorder that involves relatively rapid and fluid, but not rhythmic, limb and trunk movements. Which of the following is the most likely diagnosis?

a. Chorea gravidarum
b. Huntington's chorea
c. Alzheimer's disease
d. Multiple sclerosis
e. Amyotrophic lateral sclerosis

245. The influenza epidemic of 1918 to 1926 was associated with von Economo's encephalitis and left many persons with a syndrome indistinguishable from which of the following?

a. Sydenham's chorea
b. Alzheimer's disease
c. Multiple sclerosis
d. Amyotrophic lateral sclerosis
e. Parkinson's disease

246. A 43-year-old man has a father who died from Huntington's disease. The son was tested and found to have the gene for Huntington's disease. Which of the following is true regarding the offspring of those with Huntington's disease?

a. Half the offspring are at risk only if the affected parent is male
b. Half the offspring are at risk only if the affected parent is female
c. Half the offspring are at risk if either parent is symptomatic for the disease before the age of 30
d. Half the offspring are at risk for the disease
e. One out of four children is at risk for the disease

247. Atrophy in the head of the caudate nucleus in patients with Huntington's disease affects the shape of which of the following?

a. Cerebellum
b. Lateral ventricle
c. Third ventricle
d. Lenticular nuclei
e. Temporal lobe

248. If a patient with Huntington's disease were to be exposed to L-dopa, which of the following would most likely be evoked?

a. Generalized seizures
b. Partial seizures
c. Intention tremor
d. Scanning speech
e. Writhing and jerking movements of the limbs

249. A 26-year-old heroin addict has been using a street version of artificial heroin. The drug actually contains 1-methyl-4-phenyl-1,2,3,6-tetrahydropyridine (MPTP). The neurological syndrome for which he is at risk is clinically indistinguishable from which of the following?

a. Huntington's disease
b. Friedreich's disease
c. Sydenham's chorea
d. Parkinson's disease
e. Amyotrophic lateral sclerosis

250. A 61-year-old right-handed man presents with involuntary twitches of his left hand. He first noticed between 6 months and 1 year ago that when he is at rest, his left hand shakes. He can stop the shaking by looking at his hand and concentrating. The shaking does not impair his activities in any way. He has no trouble holding a glass of water. There is no tremor in his right hand, and his lower extremities are not affected. He has had no trouble walking, and there have been no falls. There have been no behavioral or language changes. On examination, a tremor of the left hand is evident when the man is distracted. His handwriting is mildly tremulous. He has bilateral cogwheel rigidity with contralateral activation, which is worse on the left. His rapid alternating movements are bradykinetic on the left. Which of the following is the most likely diagnosis in this case?

a. Epilepsy
b. Guillain-Barré syndrome
c. Multiple sclerosis
d. Parkinson's disease
e. Stroke

251. Which of the following brain structures are currently targets for deep brain stimulation in patients with Parkinson's disease?

a. Globus pallidus, medulla, and parietal lobe
b. Globus pallidus, subthalamic nucleus, and thalamus
c. Hippocampus, medulla, and thalamus
d. Medulla, occipital lobe, and subthalamic nucleus
e. Parietal lobe, temporal lobe, and thalamus

252. Which of the following medications is the best choice to treat Parkinson's disease?

a. Alteplase
b. Carbidopa-levodopa
c. Glatiramer
d. Interferon β-1A
e. Sertraline

253. Neurons remaining in the substantia nigra of a patient with Parkinson's disease may exhibit which of the following?

a. Intranuclear inclusion bodies
b. Intranuclear and intracytoplasmic inclusion bodies
c. Intracytoplasmic inclusion bodies
d. Neurofibrillary tangles
e. Amyloid plaques

254. A 48-year-old female psychiatric patient has parkinsonism secondary to long-term neuroleptic use. Which of the following medications might minimize her parkinsonism?

a. Trihexyphenidyl (Artane)
b. Haloperidol (Haldol)
c. Methamphetamine
d. Thioridazine (Mellaril)
e. L-dopa

255. A 70-year-old woman has 1 year of worsening gait, right-hand tremor, and rigidity. She is diagnosed with Parkinson's disease and improves dramatically with treatment. If her disease progresses, the decrement in speech that would be expected would result in which of the following?

a. Progressively inaudible speech
b. Receptive aphasia
c. Expressive aphasia
d. Word salad
e. Neologisms

256. Even though the physiologic deficiency in Parkinson's disease is of dopamine, L-dopa rather than dopamine is given to patients for which of the following reasons?

a. L-dopa induces less nausea and vomiting than dopamine
b. Dopamine is readily metabolized in the gastrointestinal tract to ineffective compounds
c. L-dopa is more readily absorbed in the gastrointestinal tract than is dopamine
d. Dopamine cannot cross the blood-brain barrier and therefore has no therapeutic effect in the CNS
e. L-dopa is more effective at dopamine receptors than is dopamine itself

257. A 25-year-old man has had motor tics since age 13. They seem to be getting worse, and now he also has involuntary obscene vocalizations. He may have largely normal behavior while being treated with which of the following?

a. L-dopa
b. Trihexyphenidyl (Artane)
c. Phenytoin (Dilantin)
d. Carbamazepine (Tegretol)
e. Haloperidol (Haldol)

258. A 72-year-old man was diagnosed with Parkinson's disease after presenting 2 years ago with asymmetric rigidity, bradykinesia, and tremor. He is being treated with carbidopa and L-dopa. Carbidopa is used in combination with L-dopa because of which of the following?

a. It has anticholinergic activity
b. It has dopaminergic activity
c. It is an antihistaminic
d. It is an antiemetic
e. It is a dopa decarboxylase inhibitor

259. After several years of successful anti-Parkinsonian treatment, a patient abruptly develops acute episodes of profound bradykinesia and rigidity. Remission of these signs occurs as abruptly as the onset. This patient probably suffers from which of the following?

a. Acute dystonia
b. Absence attacks
c. On-off phenomenon
d. Complex partial seizures
e. Drug toxicity

DIRECTIONS: Each group of questions below consists of lettered options followed by a set of numbered items. For each numbered item, select the **one** lettered option with which it is **most** closely associated. Each lettered option may be used once, more than once, or not at all.

Questions 260–263

For each clinical scenario, select the most likely condition.

a. Meigs' syndrome
b. Dopa-responsive dystonia
c. Parkinson's disease
d. Olivopontocerebellar atrophy
e. Tardive dyskinesia
f. Spasmodic torticollis
g. Whipple's disease
h. Hemifacial spasm
i. Essential tremor

260. A 53-year-old woman is unable to stop blinking forcefully, and has frequent grimacing movements of the face. At times she protrudes her tongue against her will. She has never taken any medications.

261. A 42-year-old woman has a long history of twisting movements of her head to the left. These are painful, and have resulted over the years in muscular hypertrophy affecting the sternocleidomastoid and trapezius muscles. There is no family history. The remainder of her examination is normal.

262. A 40-year-old literary agent has had worsening tremor of the hands. This has been present for 2 years, but has increasingly impaired her work ability because she is frequently required to take her clients to lunch, and she is embarrassed by her inability to eat and drink normally. A glass of wine with the meal typically helps somewhat. On exam, there is a mild head tremor, but no rest tremor of the hands. When she holds a pen by the tip at arm's length, however, a coarse tremor is readily apparent. Exam is otherwise normal.

263. A 64-year-old man has noticed dragging of the right leg and tremor and stiffness of the right hand. On exam, he has a tremor of the right hand, which disappears when he reaches to grab a pen. Movements are slower on the right than the left. He has cogwheel rigidity of the right arm.

Questions 264–268

For each clinical scenario, select the most likely diagnosis.

a. Hepatolenticular degeneration
b. Hyperparathyroidism
c. Central pontine myelinolysis
d. Akinetic mutism
e. MPTP poisoning
f. Locked-in syndrome
g. Postencephalitic parkinsonism
h. Neuroleptic effect
i. Essential tremor
j. Vegetative state
k. Hypermagnesemia
l. Rhombencephalitis

264. A 34-year-old man develops progressive depression and memory impairment over the course of 6 months. His initial neurologic evaluation reveals a metabolic acidosis associated with his dementia. His liver is firm and his spleen appears to be slightly enlarged. He has tremor and rigidity in his arms and walks with relatively little swing in his arms. His blink is substantially reduced, which gives him the appearance of staring. An MRI of the brain reveals some atrophy of the putamen and globus pallidus. His CSF is normal. His EEG is unremarkable.

265. A 19-year-old woman develops auditory hallucinations and persecutory delusions over the course of 3 days. She is hospitalized and started on haloperidol (Haldol), 2 mg three times daily. Within 1 week of treatment, she develops stooped posture and a shuffling gait. Her head is slightly tremulous and her movements are generally slowed. Her medication is changed to thioridazine (Mellaril), and trihexyphenidyl (Artane) is added. Over the next 2 weeks, she became much more animated and reports no recurrence of her hallucinations.

266. A 65-year-old man develops slurred speech, difficulty swallowing, and labored breathing over the course of 30 min. When he arrives at the emergency room, he requires ventilatory assistance. His arms and legs are flaccid, and he exhibits no voluntary movements in any of his limbs. He is able to blink his eyes when instructed and appears to have completely intact comprehension of spoken and written language. An MRI reveals extensive infarction of the ventral pons. The basilar artery is not visible on MRA.

267. A 72-year-old man requires bypass surgery to alleviate myocardial ischemia. During surgery, he has a massive myocardial infarct and protracted asystole. Resuscitative measures succeed in reestablishing a normal sinus rhythm, but postoperatively the patient remains unconscious after 48 h. Over the ensuing weeks, the patient's level of consciousness improves slightly. He appears awake at times, but does not interact in meaningful ways with visitors. He breathes independently and even swallows food when it is placed in his mouth, but he remains mute. With painful stimuli, he exhibits semipurposeful withdrawal of his limbs. His clinical status remains unchanged for several more months.

268. A 62-year-old man exhibits excessive sleepiness, slowing of movements, mild depression, and proximal muscle weakness. His proximal limb muscles are obviously atrophied. Although his blood count is normal, routine screening of serum chemistries reveals an elevated calcium level. He also has an elevated serum creatinine with reduced creatinine clearance. The patient has had abdominal discomfort intermittently for several months and has been told that his episodes of joint swelling were due to pseudogout.

Movement Disorders

Answers

244. The answer is a. (*Victor, p 78.*) Chorea gravidarum designates an involuntary movement disorder that occurs during pregnancy and involves relatively rapid and fluid, but not rhythmic, limb and trunk movements. This type of movement disorder may also appear with estrogen use, but the fundamental problem is a dramatic change in the hormonal environment of the brain. At the end of pregnancy or with the withdrawal of the offending estrogen, the movements abate. The movements that develop with chorea gravidarum may be quite asymmetric and forceful. Huntington's chorea is a progressive, uniformly fatal hereditary disease that does not fit well with the given history. The other choices are not typically characterized by this type of movement disorder.

245. The answer is e. (*Victor, p 813.*) A variety of agents can induce signs and symptoms of parkinsonism on a temporary basis, but few will evoke a persistent Parkinsonian syndrome. After the epidemic of encephalitis lethargica of 1918 to 1926, there were many cases of postencephalitic parkinsonism. The causative agent was believed to be an influenza virus, but it could not be isolated with the techniques available at the time of the epidemic. Postinfluenzal parkinsonism still develops, but the incidence is too rare to establish that this virus is the only virus capable of producing parkinsonism. Early in the infection, patients may exhibit a transient chorea. As the chorea abates, the parkinsonism appears and persists.

246. The answer is d. (*Kandel, p 865.*) Huntington's disease is transmitted in an autosomal dominant fashion. The age at which the patient becomes symptomatic is variable and has no effect on the probability of transmitting the disease. The defect underlying this degenerative disease is an abnormal expansion of a region of chromosome 4 containing a triplicate repeat (CAG) sequence. Normal individuals have between 6 and 34 copies of this CAG section; patients with Huntington's disease may have from 37 to more than 100 repeats. Once expanded beyond 40 copies, the repeats are unstable and may further increase as they are passed on from one generation to the next. An increased number of repeats leads to a phenomenon known as *anticipation,* by which successive generations have earlier disease onset.

247. The answer is b. *(Greenberg, pp 14–16.)* As the caudate atrophies, the frontal tip of the lateral ventricle becomes increasingly rhomboidal in shape. The head of the caudate is usually atrophic early in the course of Huntington's disease, and this will usually be evident by the time the patient is symptomatic, if not sooner. On MRI or CT scanning, the head of the caudate gives the frontal and parietal components of the lateral ventricle its typical comma, or boomerang, appearance.

248. The answer is e. *(Victor, p 1125.)* Writhing and jerking movements of the limbs are part of the chorea that typically develops with Huntington's disease. Dopaminergic drugs, such as L-dopa, bromocriptine, and lisuride, may unmask chorea. This is inadvisable as a diagnostic technique because it may contribute to the premature symptom of chorea. Dopamine antagonists, such as haloperidol, may be used to suppress chorea, but also carry the risk of provoking tardive dyskinesia. Huntington's disease is characterized pathologically by loss of several neuronal types in the striatum (caudate and putamen). It has been hypothesized that the occurrence of dopaminergic-induced chorea in Huntington's disease is related to increased sensitivity of the dopamine receptors in the remaining striatal neurons, although there are abnormalities in several other neurotransmitters as well. Choreiform movements develop in a variety of other conditions; the one most similar to Huntington's disease is hereditary acanthocytosis.

249. The answer is d. *(Victor, p 73.)* Young adults who have self-administered MPTP in an effort to achieve an opiate high have developed progressive damage to the substantia nigra. The neurologic syndrome that results from this damage is indistinguishable from Parkinson's disease, except that it evolves over weeks or months rather than years. Affected persons exhibit rigidity, tremor, and bradykinesia. That a toxin can produce a syndrome indistinguishable from Parkinson's disease has increased speculation that some—perhaps many—persons with Parkinson's disease have had environmental exposure to a toxin that produced degeneration of the substantia nigra.

250. The answer is d. *(Bradley pp 2132–2133.)* The tremor is of a Parkinsonian type. The patient also has the classic findings of Parkinson's disease: asymmetric tremor, rigidity, and bradykinesia. Epilepsy is characterized by repeated unprovoked seizures. Hand shaking can be the result of a focal motor seizure, but the presentation overall makes epilepsy an unlikely diagnosis. Guillain-Barré syndrome is a peripheral demyelinating disease that usually presents as an ascending motor deficit. Multiple sclerosis is a central nervous system (CNS) demyelinating disease. It presents with individual episodes of CNS deficits, which usually recover to some extent. Stroke is characterized by the acute onset of a neurological deficit due to nerve infarction. Tremor would be an exceedingly rare presentation for stroke, and it would not evolve over 6 to 12 months.

251. The answer is b. *(Bradley, pp 2138–2139.)* Current theory of Parkinson's disease pathology is based on the premise that the substantia nigra pars compacta has decreased dopamine production, which eventually leads to overinhibition of thalamocortical pathways. The thalamus may be directly intervened on to decrease this overinhibition. Alternatively, the globus pallidus interna may be lesioned or stimulated, because it directly inhibits the thalamus. A third approach is to lesion or stimulate the subthalamic nucleus, which has an excitatory connection on the globus pallidus interna and substantia nigra pars reticulata. The medulla, hippocampus, temporal lobe, and occipital lobe are not involved in this pathway.

252. The answer is b. *(Bradley, pp 2134–2138.)* Parkinson's disease symptoms are due in large part to dopamine depletion. Carbidopa-levodopa can replete dopamine and alleviate symptoms. Alteplase is used to dissolve blood clots during acute strokes or heart attacks. Glatiramer and interferon β-1A are used to treat multiple sclerosis, and have been shown to decrease attacks. Both are thought to work through immunomodulation. Sertraline is a selective serotonin reuptake inhibitor. By increasing serotonin concentrations, it is effective for the treatment of depression.

253. The answer is c. *(Bradley, p 2133)* The intracytoplasmic inclusion bodies commonly seen in patients with idiopathic Parkinson's disease are called Lewy bodies. They are eosinophilic inclusions with poorly staining halos surrounding them. They may be round or oblong in shape and are most common in the substantia nigra, locus coeruleus, and substantia innominata. They appear to consist of aggregated neurofilaments. Degenerative changes may be remarkably asymmetric in patients with Parkinson's disease.

254. The answer is a. (*Bradley, pp 2134–2135.*) Trihexyphenidyl (Artane) is an anticholinergic drug. It is presumed to decrease signs of parkinsonism caused by drugs that interfere with dopamine neurotransmission by creating a relative deficiency of acetylcholine neurotransmission. In a very simplistic view of the CNS, the cholinergic and dopaminergic systems have antagonistic actions.

255. The answer is a. (*Victor, p 1130.*) Language is not disturbed in Parkinson's disease, as it is with aphasias. It is the clarity and volume of speech that suffers. Handwriting is similarly disturbed. The patient has increasingly smaller and less legible penmanship as he or she continues to write. This is referred to as *micrographia.*

256. The answer is d. (*Victor, pp 1133–1134.*) L-dopa crosses the blood-brain barrier easily and is subsequently converted to dopamine in the CNS. Conversion of L-dopa to dopamine occurs outside the CNS in a wide variety of tissues, but once converted to dopamine in the periphery, the drug becomes inaccessible to the brain. Peripheral conversion of L-dopa to dopamine is routinely inhibited by adding a dopa decarboxylase inhibitor to the therapeutic regimen. Carbidopa, the inhibitor most widely used, does not penetrate the blood-brain barrier substantially. Because it is largely excluded from the CNS, carbidopa cannot inhibit the conversion of L-dopa to dopamine in the brain.

257. The answer is e. (*Bradley, p 2162.*) The scenario described is that associated with Tourette syndrome. The affected person is usually over 21 years of age and cannot control the obscene and scatological remarks. With Tourette syndrome there appears to be an autosomal dominant pattern of inheritance with variable penetrance. Most affected persons are men. A variety of drugs may help suppress the tics that are characteristic of this syndrome. These include haloperidol, pimozide, trifluoperazine, and fluphenazine. Antiepileptics, such as carbamazepine and phenytoin, are not useful. Trihexyphenidyl and benztropine are useful in suppressing the parkinsonism that may develop with haloperidol administration, but are not useful in the management of Tourette syndrome.

258. The answer is e. (*Bradley, pp 2134–2135.*) Dopa decarboxylase converts L-dopa to dopamine. Carbidopa crosses the blood-brain barrier poorly, and so its inhibition of this enzyme is restricted to activity outside the CNS. Conversion of L-dopa to dopamine continues to occur in the CNS when the patient takes Sinemet, a combination of L-dopa and carbidopa.

259. The answer is c. (*Victor, p 1135.*) The on-off effect is commonly seen in persons who have had Parkinson's disease for several years. Maintaining more stable levels of anti-Parkinsonian medication in the blood does not eliminate this phenomenon of abruptly worsening and remitting symptoms. Variability in the responsiveness of the CNS to the medication, rather than in the medication levels, underlies the phenomenon.

260. The answer is a. (*Victor, p 115.*) Meigs' syndrome is a form of focal dystonia characterized by blepharospasm, forceful jaw opening, lip retraction, neck contractions, and tongue thrusting. Sometimes these features are produced by phenothiazine or butyrophenone use, but they may also occur idiopathically, more often in women than men, with onset in the sixth decade. Botulinum toxin injection has been more effective in treatment than any oral medication.

261. The answer is f. (*Victor, pp 113–114.*) Spasmodic torticollis is another very common form of focal dystonia. It usually begins in early adult life. The contractions of the neck muscles may be painful and also produce hypertrophy. Standing and walking worsen the contractions, and typically a trick, or geste, such as touching the chin or resting the head against a pillow, may reduce the spasms. Spontaneous remissions may occur. Trihexiphenidyl (Artane) and a number of other medications may be used, generally without much success; effective improvement generally does not occur until botulinum toxin injections are given.

262. The answer is i. (*Victor, pp 100–103.*) Essential tremor comes on during action and remits when the limb is relaxed, unlike the tremor of Parkinson's disease. It often affects the head as well as the arms, also unlike Parkinson's disease. Patients are often very disturbed by the tremor, particularly as it leads to a great deal of social embarrassment. There is no associated slowness of activity (bradykinesia), rigidity, or cognitive disturbance. Patients frequently report improvement with alcohol, to the extent that some patients may resort to use of alcohol on a chronic basis to reduce their symptoms. Although it is often referred to as familial tremor, there is some disagreement on this point because it may simply be the case that patients with the condition are more likely to refer relatives for evaluation. Beta blockers and primidone may be used to treat this condition.

263. The answer is c. (*Victor, pp 1128–1137.*) Idiopathic Parkinson's disease is characterized by the classic combination of tremor, rigidity, bradykinesia, and postural instability. The typical tremor is a 4-Hz pill-rolling tremor, affecting one side more than the other. Action tremor may also occur. The classic pathologic hallmarks of the disease are a loss of pigmented cells in the substantia nigra and other nuclei, and the finding of the Lewy body, which is an eosinophilic cytoplasmic inclusion in the remaining cells of the substantia nigra.

264. The answer is a. (*Bradley, p 2159.*) Hepatolenticular degeneration (Wilson's disease) often becomes symptomatic in the second or third decade of life, but its initial presentation may be delayed until the fourth or fifth decade. Renal tubular acidosis develops along with hepatic fibrosis. Systemic problems include heart and lung damage, but most patients become most symptomatic from their brain and liver disease. Dementia is progressive if the patient is not treated. Hepatic disease will progress to hepatic failure if the patient is left untreated. Appropriate treatment includes the chelating agent penicillamine, which depletes the body of copper.

265. The answer is h. (*Bradley, pp 1928–1929.*) Butyrophenones, the most commonly prescribed of which is haloperidol, routinely produce some signs of parkinsonism if they are used at high doses for more than a few days. This psychotic young woman proved to be less sensitive to the Parkinsonian effects of the phenothiazine thioridazine than she was to haloperidol. Adding the anticholinergic trihexyphenidyl may also have helped to reduce the patient's parkinsonism. Another commonly used medication that can cause parkinsonism, in addition to tardive dyskinesia, is metoclopramide hydrochloride (Reglan).

266. The answer is f. (*Bradley, p 1207.*) Consciousness is preserved in the locked-in syndrome, but the patient is paralyzed from the eyes down. Survival is usually limited to days or weeks in patients with this clinical syndrome. In most cases, the locked-in syndrome develops because of ischemic or hemorrhagic damage to the pons, such as that occurring with basilar artery occlusion.

267. The answer is j. (*Bradley, p 44.*) The vegetative state is a clinical condition in which autonomic activity is sustained with little evidence of cognitive function. With protracted asystole, the patient may sustain extensive damage to the cerebral cortex with little damage to the brainstem. The ischemic damage to the cerebrum should be evident on MRI soon after the injury. This type of damage is usually responsible for the appearance of the vegetative state. It also may develop with drowning or other causes of protracted hypoxia.

268. The answer is b. (*Bradley, pp 1094, 1097, 1690.*) Primary hyperparathyroidism develops in the elderly and may be overlooked or misdiagnosed. The elevated calcium (over 11.5 mg/dL) that is characteristic of the disturbance is dismissed as an immobilization phenomenon or misconstrued as evidence of an occult neoplasm. The appearance of pseudogout should raise the probability of hyperparathyroidism substantially. The calcium level may in fact be normal when it is checked, but the parathyroid hormone levels will be elevated.

Disorders of Myelination

Questions

DIRECTIONS: Each item below contains a question followed by suggested responses. Select the **one best** response to each question.

269. A 21-year-old right-handed female student was working in the photography lab 1 week ago, which required standing all day. After that, she experienced a cold sensation in the left foot and her entire left leg fell asleep. The feeling lasted 4 to 5 days and then slowly went away. Her right lower extremity was fine. Coughing, sneezing, and the Valsalva maneuver did not worsen her symptoms. She had a slight back pain, which she thought was due to using a poor mattress. Past history includes an episode of optic neuritis in the left eye 2 years ago. At that time, she was reportedly depressed and was sleeping constantly. One day, her left eye became blurred and her vision went out. In 1 week, her vision returned to normal. Her vision now is 20/20. She has not had a repeat episode since then. She had an MRI of her brain, which was normal at that time. She drinks alcohol occasionally and does not use any illicit drugs. Her only medication is birth control pills. Examination is significant for brisk reflexes and sustained clonus at the right ankle. Babinski sign is present on the right. Testing is positive for oligoclonal bands. Which of the following is the most likely diagnosis in this case?

a. Seizure
b. Transient ischemic attack
c. Anaplastic astrocytoma
d. Multiple sclerosis
e. Parkinson's disease

270. A patient has brought some test results from an outside doctor with her today. One of the results indicates that oligoclonal bands were positive. What are oligoclonal bands?

a.   Wave frequency changes on the EEG during sleep
b.   Markings about the iris
c.   Pathologic features of Alzheimer's disease
d.   Chromosomal markings found with multiple sclerosis (MS)
e.   Immunoglobulin patterns in the CSF with MS

271. A 39-year-old woman with multiple sclerosis has bladder spasticity and clonus of the lower extremities. On briskly flexing her neck forward, which of the following is she most likely to report?

a.   Dystonic posturing of the legs
b.   An electrical sensation radiating down the spine or into the legs
c.   Bilateral wristdrop
d.   Spontaneous evacuation of the bladder and bilateral extensor plantar responses
e.   Rapidly evolving hemifacial pain

272. A 19-year-old man had an episode of left optic neuritis, which resolved over several weeks. Two years later there was a monthlong episode of bladder dysfunction. The patient underwent many tests and was told that he had multiple sclerosis. The CSF in persons with multiple sclerosis will typically exhibit which of the following?

a.   Glucose content of less than 20% of the serum content
b.   Persistently elevated total protein content
c.   Persistently elevated immunoglobulin G (IgG) content
d.   Mononuclear cell counts of greater than 100 cells per μL
e.   Erythrocyte counts of greater than 10 cells per μL

273. A 35-year-old man with multiple sclerosis initially presented 4 years ago with left eye optic neuritis. He did not receive steroids at that time. Two years ago he had loss of sensation in his hands that progressed over weeks to motor involvement, limiting his ability to write with the left hand. He received steroids at that time. Four years ago, he began interferon β-1A. One year ago, he developed right leg weakness, constipation, and urinary urgency. He received steroids at that time as well. He now presents with symptoms that concern him about the possible start of a new flare. Two days ago, he noticed decreased sensation in the palm of his right hand that is worse when he exercises. This has gotten a little worse over the past 2 days. Yesterday, he noticed diminished sensation along the lower right trunk in the front and back. He has no pain, tingling, exacerbation of symptoms with neck movement, neck injury, incontinence, gait disturbance, diplopia, fever, chills, nausea, or vomiting. Examination findings include full visual fields with a left afferent pupillary defect. Bulk, strength, and tone are normal. Light touch is decreased over the left trunk and back over roughly the T8 to T12 dermatomes. Finger tapping, rapid alternating movements, finger-nose-finger, and heel tapping to shin are normal. Which of the following is the most appropriate pharmacological treatment for this patient at this time?

a. Interferon β-1B
b. Corticosteroids
c. Gabapentin
d. Glatiramer
e. Pramipexole

274. Multiple sclerosis is the most common demyelinating disease in the United States, affecting approximately one person in how many?

a. 100
b. 500
c. 1000
d. 5000
e. 10,000

275. A patient with suspected multiple sclerosis undergoes multimodality evoked potentials, EEG, MRI, and CSF testing. Which of the following evoked response patterns is most often abnormal in patients with early MS?

a. Brainstem auditory evoked response (BAER)
b. Far-field somatosensory evoked response (SSER)
c. Visual evoked response (VER)
d. Jolly test
e. Sensory nerve conduction test

276. A 37-year-old woman with progressive multiple sclerosis is being admitted for intravenous glucocorticoid therapy. She was diagnosed with multiple sclerosis 10 years ago after presenting with bilateral decreased visual acuity. She had an abnormal MRI at that time. She has been hospitalized approximately nine times since presentation, with her flares commonly consisting of increasing bilateral lower extremity weakness and decreased sensation manifested as a heavy feeling, waxing and waning generalized fatigue, bilateral hand tingling, and occasional nondescript speech changes that make her sound as though she has a slight accent. She has also had bilateral optic neuritis and one transient episode of aphasia in the past. She was last hospitalized 3 years ago. For the past 2 years she has been on cyclophosphamide and methylprednisolone, originally every 4 weeks, and now every 6 weeks, with the last treatment 1 month ago. She has tried and failed interferon β therapy. For the 2 months prior to admission, the patient has had worsening bilateral lower extremity weakness/heaviness, increased fatigue, and mild low back numbness, as well as intermittent and alternating decreased hearing in both ears at work. She has also noticed mild unsteadiness when walking. Which of the following should be included among her admission orders?

a. Heart-healthy diet
b. Ranitidine 150 mg bid
c. Neurological checks every hour for the first 48 h
d. Placement of central venous line
e. Stat head CT for change in mental status

277. A 29-year-old man contracted HIV-1 through homosexual activity 5 years ago. He had been doing well on HAART, but stopped taking his medications 8 months ago because he thought that he would be better off. Two months ago he was successfully treated for *Pneumocystis carinii* pneumonia. A papovavirus infection of the central nervous system (CNS) in this person would be most likely to produce which of the following?

a. Adrenoleukodystrophy
b. Multiple sclerosis
c. Subacute sclerosing panencephalitis (SSPE)
d. Progressive multifocal leukoencephalopathy (PML)
e. Metachromatic leukodystrophy

278. A 3-month-old child has a rapid regression of psychomotor function and loss of sight. There is increased urinary excretion of N-acetyl-L-aspartic acid. A preliminary diagnosis of Canavan's disease (Canavan-van Bogaert-Bertrand disease; spongy degeneration of infancy) is made. This is a demyelinating disease that produces retardation in infants, is inherited in an autosomal recessive pattern, and results in which of the following?

a. Anencephaly
b. Microcephaly
c. Porencephaly
d. Macrocephaly
e. Dolichocephaly

279. A 58-year-old man with a basilar tip aneurysm is referred by a neurosurgeon. He has a 4-year history of progressive spastic paraparesis. He has recently had urge incontinence of urine. He also has numbness in the right toes more than the left, and pain in the thighs and back. There have been some gradual fluctuations, but no clear, discrete episodes of deterioration. He has had no disturbances of vision, eye movement, or motor control of the upper extremities. He was referred when surgical clipping of the aneurysm 3 months ago failed to help his symptoms. Which of the following is the most appropriate next diagnostic test?

a. Cerebral angiography
b. Spinal angiography
c. MRI of the spinal cord
d. Spinal cord biopsy
e. VER

280. Cystometrographic analysis of bladder function in a patient with long-term multiple sclerosis is likely to show which of the following abnormalities?

a. Bladder hypotonia
b. Large residual volume of urine
c. Premature bladder emptying
d. Good voluntary control of bladder emptying
e. Urinary tract infection

281. A patient with multiple sclerosis has worsening leg weakness. He has severe spasms of his legs bilaterally, and is increasingly unable to ambulate because of this. A reasonable symptomatic treatment option would be which of the following?

a. Cyclophosphamide
b. Baclofen
c. Gabapentin
d. Amitriptyline hydrochloride
e. Propranolol

282. You are counseling a 22-year-old woman with the recent diagnosis of multiple sclerosis. She wants to know what if any lifestyle changes she may have to make. Which of the following factors might be expected to worsen multiple sclerosis symptoms?

a. Bright lights
b. Red wine
c. Tyramine-containing compounds
d. Hot weather
e. Amantadine

DIRECTIONS: Each group of questions below consists of lettered options followed by a set of numbered items. For each numbered item, select the **one** lettered option with which it is **most** closely associated. Each lettered option may be used once, more than once, or not at all.

Questions 283–288

For each patient, select the most likely diagnosis.

a. Neuromyelitis optica (Devic's disease)
b. Central pontine myelinolysis
c. Marchiafava-Bignami disease
d. Acute disseminated encephalomyelitis
e. Pelizaeus-Merzbacher disease
f. Leber's optic atrophy
g. Alexander's disease
h. Adrenoleukodystrophy
i. Canavan's disease

283. A 23-year-old woman awakens with bilateral leg weakness and numbness, urinary retention, and impaired bowel control. She has had several episodes of blurred vision over the previous 2 years, but these had always been attributed to idiopathic papillitis.

284. Two weeks after recovering from a febrile illness associated with a productive cough, a 19-year-old man complains of headache and neck stiffness. These complaints are associated with fever and are soon followed by deteriorating cognitive function. He becomes disoriented, lethargic, and increasingly unresponsive. MRI reveals widespread damage to the white matter of the cerebral hemispheres.

285. A 24-year-old man has progressive loss of vision over the course of 5 years. A visual field examination reveals a centrocecal scotoma. Two of his cousins have similar problems with visual loss. Both of the affected relatives are male and in their twenties. Genetic testing reveals a mutation of mitochondrial DNA.

286. Two brothers, 4 and 7 years of age, exhibit limb ataxia, nystagmus, and mental retardation. MRI of their brains reveals areas of abnormal signal in the white matter. Cerebellar involvement is substantial. Both boys also have abnormally low serum cortisol levels.

287. A 3-month-old boy exhibits nystagmus and limb tremors unassociated with seizures. Over the next few years, he develops optic atrophy, choreoathetotic limb movements, seizures, and gait ataxia. He dies during status epilepticus and at autopsy is found to have widespread myelin breakdown with myelin preservation in islands about the blood vessels. The pathologist diagnoses a sudanophilic leukodystrophy to describe the pattern of staining observed on slides prepared to look for myelin breakdown products.

288. A 54-year-old alcoholic man is brought to the emergency room with profound agitation. He is believed to have delirium tremens and is treated with thiamine and intravenous fluids. His serum sodium is noted to be markedly depressed, and intravenous supplements are adjusted to rapidly correct this hyponatremia. He becomes acutely quadriplegic and unresponsive and dies within 24 h.

Disorders of Myelination

Answers

269. The answer is d. (*Victor, pp 961–962.*) This is a typical history for multiple sclerosis (MS). Multiple sclerosis is a progressive demyelinating disease of the central nervous system. Risk factors include a first-time demyelinating episode such as optic neuritis. Patients are more commonly in the 20 to 30 age range, with a higher incidence in women. A transient ischemic attack is a brief period of brain ischemia causing neurological deficits that resolve within 24 h. Patients who have a transient ischemic attack are at increased risk for stroke. A seizure is abnormal rhythmic electrical brain activity with a clinical correlation. There is nothing in the history to suggest that this patient had a seizure or a seizure predisposing factor. Seizure predisposing factors include previous seizure, brain trauma, brain hemorrhage, and encephalitis. An anaplastic astrocytoma is a malignant high-grade brain tumor. These often present with a seizure or hemorrhage. Risk factors include previous brain tumor. Parkinson's disease is caused by a loss of dopaminergic neurons. It is characterized by asymmetric slowness, rigidity, and tremor. Risk factors include family history.

270. The answer is e. (*Victor, p 969.*) Between 85 and 90% of patients with MS exhibit oligoclonal banding on electrophoretic studies of their CSF. This limited number of bands of excess immunoglobulin indicates that the species of IgG produced by the disease fall into a relatively small number of families. The proteins are not highly diverse, as would be the case with a polyclonal gammopathy.

271. The answer is b. (*Victor, p 962.*) The peculiar sensory phenomenon in which the patient feels an electrical sensation radiating down the spine when the neck is passively flexed is called Lhermitte's sign and is believed to signify spinal cord disease. Patients with MS who have little more than optic atrophy and no evidence of spinal cord involvement may report the sensation. Dystonic posturing may also occur in patients with MS, but the posturing is usually spontaneous. A massive Babinski response may produce bladder evacuation and extensor plantar responses as well as involuntary leg withdrawal in these same patients. This type of reflex response is usually elicited by stimuli to the feet or legs rather than by manipulation of the neck or spine.

272. The answer is c. *(Bradley, pp 1650–1651.)* The IgG content of the CSF remains elevated even between acute exacerbations of the MS. The IgG has a distinctive κ light chain composition. This immunoglobulin typically accounts for more than 15% of the total protein content in the CSF of the patient with MS.

273. The answer is b. *(Victor, p 973.)* Corticosteroids are an appropriate treatment for a multiple sclerosis flare. They will reduce the length and severity of the flare in most cases, although they are not likely to change the long-term disease outcome. Interferon β-IB and glatiramer are appropriate treatments to reduce the frequency of multiple sclerosis flares; however, they are not useful for the acute treatment of a flare. Gabapentin is an anticonvulsant medication that is also useful for the treatment of neuropathic pain, such as burning and allodynia. It will not help a multiple sclerosis flare. Pramipexole is a dopamine agonist used to treat parkinsonism. It has no role in the treatment of multiple sclerosis.

274. The answer is c. *(Bradley, pp 1636–1638.)* Approximately 250,000 people in the United States carry the diagnosis of MS. Most of the affected persons live in northern states, but no state is exempt from reports of MS. Because there is no test to unequivocally establish the diagnosis, the exact number of active cases in the United States can be approximated only very roughly.

275. The answer is c. *(Bradley, p 1651.)* Optic neuritis occurs early and often in many patients with MS. This involves inflammation and demyelination of the optic nerve and slows conduction along the optic nerve. Components of the VER may be slowed or even absent. That an evoked response is disturbed is not proof that the patient has MS, as any problem that produces optic neuritis will disturb the VER. The Jolly test is an evoked response involving muscles. A peripheral nerve is shocked at 5 to 15 times per second, and the pattern of action potentials elicited in the muscle innervated is recorded. Sensory nerve conduction studies also involve an evoked response to a shock, with the resulting signal tracked in the sensory nerve stimulated. Muscle and peripheral nerve function is typically normal in patients with MS, unless they have an unrelated disease of the peripheral nervous system.

276. The answer is b. *(Kasper, p 2466.)* Gastric disturbances are a possible side effect of corticosteroid use. Ranitidine is an appropriate prophylactic treatment. Patients with high cholesterol should be given a heart-healthy diet. Neurological checks every hour, central venous line, and stat head CT for change in mental status are all things that should be done for unstable trauma patients with a cranial component.

277. The answer is d. *(Bradley, pp 1594–1596.)* Adrenoleukodystrophy, MS, SSPE, PML, and metachromatic leukodystrophy are all demyelinating diseases, but PML is the only one confidently linked to a virus. The specific strains of papovavirus most often implicated in PML are BK, JC, and SV40. The patients at risk for this often lethal demyelinating process are those with lymphomas, leukemias, and AIDS. Patients on immunosuppressants face substantially lower risk, but are at higher risk than the general population.

278. The answer is d. *(Victor, pp 1000–1001.)* Canavan's disease may produce developmental regression at about 6 months of age. The infant develops extensor posturing and rigidity. Myoclonic seizures may develop. Underlying the disease is a defect in N-acetylaspartic acid metabolism. Elevated levels of this material can be detected in the blood and urine, but elevated levels in the brain establish the diagnosis. Changes in brain white matter are widespread and may result in a spongiform appearance. There is an increase in brain volume and weight.

279. The answer is c. *(Bradley, pp 1647–1649.)* This patient has a gradually progressive myelopathy. The differential diagnosis is broad, but MS is high on the list. A subset of patients with MS consists of middle-aged men with a progressive form of the disease. An MRI of the spinal cord could show MS plaques in the cord or other abnormalities intrinsic to the spinal cord parenchyma, and could also exclude compressive lesions. Vascular malformations of the spinal cord can also be seen in this way, although sometimes spinal angiography is required for definitive diagnosis. Cerebral angiography would not be helpful, except to evaluate for residual aneurysm, which is unlikely to be related to this patient's problem. Spinal cord biopsy is unwarranted in this case unless a specific indication is provided on neuroimaging. Visual evoked responses may be abnormal in MS, even without clinical evidence of disease, but would not account for the patient's spastic paraparesis.

280. The answer is c. (*Bradley, p 426.*) Patients with a multiple sclerosis often develop a spastic (upper motor neuron) bladder. There is little or no residual urine in the bladder after emptying because bladder contractility is good, but distensibility is poor. The bladder does not distend substantially because of corticospinal tract disease, which produces spasticity. The patient usually has urgency or incontinence.

281. The answer is b. (*Bradley, p 1654.*) Baclofen is an antispasmodic agent that may be used in MS. Additional agents that may be used include tiazidine or benzodiazepines. Cyclophosphamide is an immunosuppressive drug that may be used to treat MS, but would not be considered a symptomatic therapy.

282. The answer is d. (*Bradley, p 1642.*) Patients with demyelinating diseases often notice that their symptoms become worse in conditions of increased temperature. In fact, one old way of diagnosing MS called for the patient to be submerged in a tub of warm water; if the deficits worsened, this was considered a sign of MS. This heat sensitivity, also called Uhthoff's phenomenon, explains why patients often feel worse in the summer or on taking hot showers. MS should be considered when seeing a patient who notices exercise-induced symptoms, because the increased heat that is generated by exercise may be enough to exacerbate the deficits.

283. The answer is a. (*Victor, pp 966–967.*) Neuromyelitis optica produces signs and symptoms of bilateral optic neuritis in association with a transverse myelitis. The paraparesis, bladder and bowel dysfunction, and sensory deficit signal a transverse myelitis—that is, an inflammatory demyelinating lesion that transects much of the spinal cord. In some cases, the pathology shows a necrotizing process in the spinal cord. All of these problems may develop with MS, but cerebellar involvement, more scattered cerebral involvement, and a generally less circumscribed pattern of deficits are more likely. Adults are especially likely to develop a pattern more typical of relapsing-remitting MS after an initial episode of neuromyelitis optica. Children presenting with neuromyelitis optica may have no other signs or symptoms of demyelination.

284. The answer is d. *(Victor, pp 975–978.)* Acute disseminated encephalomyelitis is often fatal. On examination of the brain, damage to small blood vessels and to perivascular tissues in the white matter of the cerebral hemispheres is extensive and coalescent. The diagnosis is suggested by the MRI or CT picture of rapidly evolving white matter damage associated with a high erythrocyte sedimentation rate (ESR) and a cerebrospinal fluid (CSF) under increased pressure with elevated red cell and white cell counts and elevated protein content. The CSF glucose content is usually normal.

285. The answer is f. *(Victor, pp 1164–1165.)* The optic neuritis of MS produces enlargement of the physiologic blind spot, but rarely to the point where it impinges on central vision. When the blind spot extends into central vision, it is called a *centrocecal scotoma*. A young man presenting with this pattern of visual loss is much more likely to have Leber's optic atrophy or another cause of optic atrophy (e.g., tobacco-alcohol amblyopia, tertiary syphilis, or vitamin deficiencies) than to have multiple sclerosis. That other men in the family are similarly affected supports the diagnosis of the hereditary Leber's optic atrophy. This condition is caused by one of several possible mutations in mitochondrial DNA.

286. The answer is h. *(Victor, pp 1034–1036.)* Adrenal dysfunction in association with a progressive degenerative disease of the white matter suggests adrenoleukodystrophy. Some types are X-linked defects, and the fact that two brothers are affected in similar ways suggests that they have the X-linked form of adrenoleukodystrophy. X-linked adrenoleukodystrophy produces rapidly evolving brain damage in male infants or boys, with survival from onset of symptoms usually limited to 3 years. The underlying defect in this X-linked disorder is an ATP-binding transporter in the peroxisomal system responsible for long-chain fatty acid metabolism. Long-chain fatty acids accumulate in adrenal cortical and other cells. Pathophysiologically similar to, but otherwise distinct from, adrenoleukodystrophy is adrenomyeloneuropathy. It may develop in heterozygous women and usually involves less pronounced damage to the brain and more obvious damage to the spinal cord and peripheral nerves. Persons with adrenomyeloneuropathy routinely develop spastic paraparesis, problems with bladder and bowel control, and sensory disturbances in the legs.

287. The answer is e. *(Victor, p 1000.)* Pelizaeus-Merzbacher disease is a demyelinating disorder that belongs to a group of degenerative diseases known as sudanophilic leukodystrophies. Leukodystrophy refers to the disturbance of white matter, and sudanophilic refers to the Sudan staining characteristics of the involved white matter. Children with Pelizaeus-Merzbacher disease typically become symptomatic during the first months of life, but survival may extend into the third decade of life. Most affected persons are male.

288. The answer is b. *(Victor, pp 1193–1195.)* Rapid correction of hyponatremia in an alcoholic may precipitate central pontine myelinolysis (CPM), a rapidly fatal, demyelinating disorder of the brainstem. With CPM there is demyelination in the basis pontis. The destruction of myelin sheaths is usually quite symmetric and appears to begin in the median raphe. There is no inflammation associated with the demyelination, even though the changes occur acutely and progress rapidly. Death usually occurs within days or weeks of the first signs of neurologic disease. Affected persons often have hypokalemia, hypochloremia, and hypomagnesemia as well as hyponatremia. Many have a low serum osmolality associated with a normal urine osmolality, findings consistent with the syndrome of inappropriate antidiuretic hormone (SIADH). The signs of CPM may be similar to those occurring with Wernicke's encephalopathy (i.e., disturbed ocular motor function, gait disturbances, and altered consciousness and cognition). That this patient did not have Wernicke's encephalopathy was suggested by his having received thiamine before the administration of intravenous solutions, a measure usually sufficient to reduce or eliminate the risk of Wernicke's encephalopathy.

Developmental and Hereditary Disorders

Questions

DIRECTIONS: Each item below contains a question followed by suggested responses. Select the **one best** response to each question.

289. In abetalipoproteinemia, chylomicrons, very-low-density lipoprotein (VLDL), and low-density lipoprotein (LDL) are largely absent in the serum as a consequence of a mutation in which gene?

a.   Microsomal triglyceride transfer protein (MTP)
b.   Huntingtin
c.   Amyloid precursor protein
d.   Dystrophin
e.   Transfer RNA (tRNA)

290. A newborn infant has a cystic swelling at the base of the spine that is covered with hyperpigmented skin and some coarse hair. Which of the following is the most likely explanation?

a.   Mongolian spot
b.   Spina bifida occulta
c.   Nevus flammeus
d.   Meningocele
e.   Encephalocele

291. A 26-year-old man diagnosed with von Hippel-Lindau syndrome has a postcontrast computed tomography (CT) scan that reveals a cyst and two smaller masses in the left cerebellar hemisphere. Which of the following is the best recommendation to this patient?

a. Submit to surgical resection of the cerebellar lesions as soon as possible
b. Submit to radiation therapy of the cerebellar lesions immediately
c. Have follow-up MRI to look for involution of the lesions
d. Have a diagnostic lumbar puncture to look for evidence of parasitic infestation of the brain
e. Have a needle biopsy of the cerebellum to establish the histology of the cystic lesion

292. In Hirschsprung's disease, neural crest cells fail to migrate normally early in fetal development and produce potentially fatal complications within months of birth because which of the following is disturbed?

a. Intestinal motility
b. Bladder control
c. Swallowing
d. Bile secretion
e. Cardiac rhythms

Questions 293–294

293. In the tomogram below showing the base of the skull, which of the following is true regarding the first cervical vertebra?

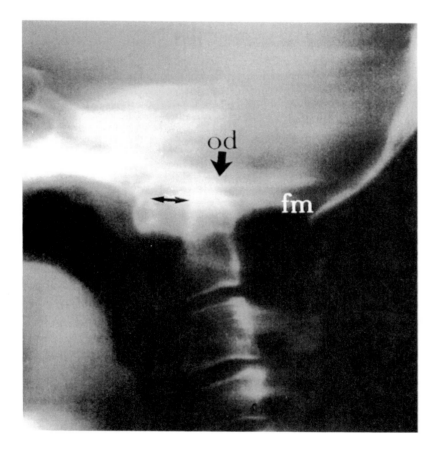

a. It is unremarkable
b. It is fused to the base of the skull
c. It is completely absent
d. It is displaced dorsally
e. It is incorporated into the odontoid process (od)

294. In the preceding x-ray, the second cervical vertebra extends above the level of the foramen magnum and places the patient at high risk of having which of the following?

a.   A meningoencephalocele
b.   A myelomeningocele
c.   Syringobulbia
d.   Syringomyelia
e.   Brainstem compression

295. Which of the following is true regarding women carrying chromosomes for fragile X syndrome?

a.   They are invariably normal
b.   They have mild retardation in about one-half of cases
c.   They have high-arched palates and hypotelorism
d.   They have hyperextensible joints
e.   They have prominent thumbs

296. A 35-year-old woman has prenatal testing done. The testing reveals that her child will have phenylketonuria (PKU). With PKU, serum may exhibit dangerously high levels of which of the following?

a.   Creatine phosphokinase (CPK)
b.   Nicotinamide
c.   Phenylketone
d.   Lactate dehydrogenase
e.   Phenylalanine

297. A diagnosis of metachromatic leukodystrophy can usually be made on the basis of which of the following?

a.   MRI
b.   Nerve biopsy
c.   Red blood cell (RBC) morphology
d.   Cerebrospinal fluid (CSF) cell morphology
e.   Electroencephalography (EEG)

298. Hepatosplenomegaly is most likely with which of the following diseases?

a. Tay-Sachs disease
b. Niemann-Pick disease
c. Alpers' disease
d. Subacute necrotizing encephalopathy
e. Wilson's disease (hepatolenticular degeneration)

299. A 25-year-old woman with epilepsy is taking divalproex sodium during the first trimester of pregnancy. She is at increased risk of having children with which of the following?

a. Holoprosencephaly
b. Defects of neural tube closure
c. Medulloblastoma
d. Agenesis of the corpus callosum
e. Kallmann syndrome

300. With agenesis of the corpus callosum, magnetic resonance imaging (MRI) will reveal which of the following?

a. Atrophy of the frontal lobes
b. Abnormally shaped lateral and third ventricles
c. Cerebellar aplasia
d. Schizencephaly
e. Encephaloclastic porencephaly

301. A boy has the onset of difficulty walking at 16 months. Reflexes are decreased. Over the course of several months, the patient becomes dysarthric and mental functioning decreases. Testing reveals that the patient has a deficiency of arylsulfatase A. Which of the following is the most likely diagnosis?

a. Sandhoff's disease
b. Tay-Sachs disease
c. Gaucher's disease
d. Metachromatic leukodystrophy
e. McArdle's disease

302. A 4-year-old previously healthy girl develops an intermittent red, scaly rash over her face, neck, hands, and legs. This is followed by developmental delay, emotional lability, and episodic cerebellar ataxia. She is diagnosed with Hartnup's disease. Her condition may respond to large supplementary doses of which of the following?

a. Vitamin C
b. Nicotinamide
c. Thiamine
d. Pyridoxine
e. α tocopherol

303. A 15-year-old boy has moderate mental retardation, attention deficit disorder, a long face, enlarged ears, and macroorchidism. Development has been steady but always at a delayed pace. Which of the following is the most likely cause for this patient's low intelligence?

a. Turner syndrome
b. Klinefelter syndrome
c. Fragile X syndrome
d. Reye syndrome
e. Tuberous sclerosis

304. A 5-year-old boy has mental retardation, homonymous hemianopsia, and hemiparesis. He had infantile spasm and still has epilepsy. Head CT reveals calcifications in the cerebral cortex in a railroad track pattern. Which of the following does this child most likely have?

a. Glioblastoma multiforme
b. Oligodendroglioma
c. Acoustic schwannoma
d. Craniopharyngioma
e. Sturge-Weber syndrome

305. A 35-year-old man has stumbling and slurred speech. His symptoms started several months ago and have progressed slowly but consistently. On neurologic examination, he is found to have scanning speech, nystagmus, limb dysmetria, and kinetic tremor. His intellectual function is normal. Which of the following is the most appropriate initial investigation?

a. Lumbar puncture
b. Serum drug screen
c. Routine urinalysis
d. Posterior fossa myelogram
e. Precontrast CT scan

306. A 29-year-old woman has progressive gait disorder and dysmetria. Laboratory studies include a hematocrit of 55% and a routine urinalysis, which reveals excess protein and some RBCs in the urine. Urine culture is negative. The initial physical examination reveals an enlarged liver and spleen. Additional physical findings will most likely include which of the following?

a. A Kayser-Fleischer ring around the cornea
b. Hypopigmented (ash-leaf) spots on the trunk
c. Telangiectasias in the fundi on retinal examination
d. Bilateral hearing loss
e. Generalized hyporeflexia

307. At age 5, a child is noted to have the loss of ankle jerks. At age 10, limb ataxia develops, followed by a peripheral neuropathy. During adolescence, retinitis pigmentosa develops. Acanthocytosis is present. These are all characteristic of which of the following?

a. Multiple sclerosis (MS)
b. Sickle cell disease
c. Abetalipoproteinemia
d. Progressive multifocal leukoencephalopathy (PML)
e. HIV subacute encephalomyelitis

308. Tuberous sclerosis is inherited in which of the following patterns?

a. A sex-linked recessive pattern
b. An autosomal dominant pattern
c. An autosomal recessive pattern
d. A pattern most consistent with newly arising mutations
e. A pattern suggesting a mitochondrial gene defect

309. An infant has a head CT performed because of a large head and failure to thrive. The diagnosis of hydrocephalus is made. Congenital hydrocephalus may develop as a consequence of which of the following first-trimester maternal disorders?

a. Complicated migraine
b. Viral infection
c. Pseudotumor cerebri
d. Chorea gravidarum
e. Intervertebral disk herniation

310. Uncorrected congenital hydrocephalus will usually produce which of the following?

a. Dolichocephaly
b. Brachycephaly
c. Holoprosencephaly
d. Macrocephaly
e. Microcephaly

311. A 6-month-old child has head lag, tongue fasciculations, and bilateral abducens palsies. MRI scan reveals a type 2 Chiari malformation. Which of the following defects would this child be likely to have?

a. A renal cyst
b. Pulmonary atelectasis
c. Spina bifida
d. Holoprosencephaly
e. A hepatic cyst

312. A 7-year-old boy is taken by his parents to see a dermatologist. They have noticed nodules on his face and are concerned. The dermatologist tells them that their child has adenoma sebaceum. Adenoma sebaceum of the face is especially common with which of the following diseases?

a. Neurofibromatosis
b. Sturge-Weber syndrome
c. Tuberous sclerosis
d. Ataxia telangiectasia
e. Fragile X syndrome

313. Within 6 years of his initial visit, a patient with von Hippel-Lindau syndrome returns with a pathologic fracture of his spine. Biopsy reveals metastatic cancer. Which of the following is the source of the tumor?

a. Cerebral hemisphere
b. Cerebellar hemisphere
c. Liver
d. Kidney
e. Spleen

314. Which of the following retinal problems tend to occur in people with tuberous sclerosis?

a. Retinal phakomas
b. Retinitis pigmentosa
c. Retinal telangiectasias
d. Retinoblastomas
e. Retinal problems are generally not part of the disease

315. Calcifications evident on the skull x-ray or CT scan of a patient with tuberous sclerosis usually represent which of the following?

a. Calcified subependymal glial nodules
b. Calcified meningeal adhesions
c. Meningeal psammoma bodies
d. Calcified astrocytomas
e. Calcified granulomas

316. A 50-year-old man presenting with "dizziness" is found to have a cyst occupying 50% of his posterior fossa and incomplete fusion of the cerebellar elements inferiorly. There is no evidence of an obstructive hydrocephalus. His longevity can be estimated to be which of the following?

a. Less than 3 months
b. Less than 1 year
c. Less than 5 years
d. Less than 10 years
e. Unaffected by this finding

317. Which of the following is the treatment of choice for children with infantile spasms?

a. Carbamazepine (Tegretol)
b. Phenobarbital
c. Phenytoin (Dilantin)
d. Divalproex sodium (Depakote)
e. Adrenocorticotropic hormone (ACTH)

318. A 9-year-old boy has been generally healthy. However, his parents are concerned that his many areas of hyperpigmented skin may have some significance. They have been told that these are café au lait spots. Café au lait spots are commonly found on patients with which of the following diseases?

a. Tuberous sclerosis
b. Neurofibromatosis
c. MS
d. Sturge-Weber syndrome
e. Ataxia telangiectasia

319. The newborn infant with motor neuron disease is likely to exhibit which of the following?

a. Seizures
b. Hypotonia
c. Hypsarrhythmia
d. Moro reflexes
e. Spina bifida

320. Many children with Tay-Sachs disease develop blindness before they die, with retinal accumulation of gangliosides that produces which of the following?

a. Optic neuritis
b. Cherry red spots
c. Chorioretinitis
d. Retinal detachments
e. Waxy exudates

321. The parents of a 10-year-old boy bring their child in to see you. The child has been diagnosed with cerebral palsy, and the parents do not really understand what this means. As part of your explanation, which of the following would you tell them?

a. Cerebral palsy is a static encephalopathy because deficits do not appear after birth
b. Cerebral palsy is a static encephalopathy because the injury to the brain does not progress
c. Cerebral palsy is a static encephalopathy because affected persons fail to reach any developmental milestones on time
d. Cerebral palsy is a static encephalopathy because affected persons have resting tremors
e. Cerebral palsy is a static encephalopathy because the EEG exhibits a disorganized background rhythm

322. A 6-year-old child is brought to the neurologist because of developmental delay. Her morphological features are typical and chromosome analysis confirms a diagnosis of Down syndrome (trisomy 21). The brain of this patient is expected to have which of the following characteristics?

a. Smaller than normal for age and body size
b. Larger than normal for age and body size
c. Abnormally long in anteroposterior measurements
d. Hydrocephalic
e. Excessively convoluted

323. Porencephaly usually develops as a consequence of which of the following?

a. Fetal alcohol syndrome
b. Vascular or other destructive injuries to the fetal brain
c. Trisomy 13
d. Trisomy 21
e. Dandy-Walker syndrome

324. What percentage of patients with tuberous sclerosis have mental retardation?

a. 1
b. 10
c. 25
d. 65
e. 99

325. A child is born to a 19-year-old woman who has had two to eight drinks per day throughout her pregnancy. What is the major pathologic effect of alcohol on the central nervous system of the developing fetus?

a. Cerebral ischemia
b. Periventricular hemorrhage
c. Macrocephaly
d. Impaired neuronal migration
e. Holoprosencephaly

326. A 37-year-old man has an MRI performed by his primary care doctor because of a long history of headaches. It is notable only for the finding of a type 1 Chiari malformation. He is sent to a neurologist for further evaluation. A type 1 Chiari malformation usually becomes symptomatic as which of the following in adults?

a. Epilepsy
b. Hydrocephalus
c. Ataxia
d. Dementia
e. Psychosis

327. A 25-year-old mother develops an illness during pregnancy. A diagnosis of cytomegalovirus (CMV) infection is made by serology. Prenatal CMV infections may produce which retinal disturbance?

a. Chorioretinitis
b. Cherry red spot
c. Microaneurysms
d. Hypervascularity
e. Hemorrhage

Developmental and Hereditary Disorders

Answers

289. The answer is a. (*Bradley p 2336.*) This disorder appears to be due to a mutation in the gene that encodes a subunit of the MTP, which results in impaired VLDL formation and consequent decreased vitamin E delivery to the peripheral and central nervous system. In addition to an abnormal plasma lipid profile, patients have disturbed fat absorption. Presumably, it is the disturbed lipid that deforms the erythrocyte cell wall, but erythrocyte production levels are relatively normal. Fat is increased in the liver, and patients exhibit lactose intolerance. Central nervous system amyloid collections develop in Alzheimer's disease.

290. The answer is d. (*Victor, p 1062.*) The Mongolian spot is a benign discoloration of the newborn's skin at the base of the spine. It is usually oval, well circumscribed, flat, and slightly hyperpigmented or otherwise discolored. Spina bifida occulta is a defect in the superior elements of the spinal column that is unassociated with meningeal or spinal cord abnormalities. It may be evidenced superficially by a dimple in the skin or a tuft of hair overlying the base of the spine. When there is evagination of the meninges (dura mater and pia arachnoid) about the cord or cauda equina through the defect in the spine, the condition is called a *meningocele*. Extrusion of meningeal and neural elements together is called a *meningomyelocele*. An encephalocele is a defect in the skull with extrusion of brain. Nevus flammeus is a congenital port-wine spot, usually developing on the face.

291. The answer is a. (*Swaiman, pp 539–540.*) The cystic lesion and the other cerebellar lesions are most likely hemangioblastomas. These hemangioblastomas often bleed and produce potentially lethal intracranial hematomas. Radiation therapy and needle biopsies would increase the risk of bleeding. Rather than spontaneously involuting, these lesions generally enlarge and become more unstable as time passes. Intracerebellar hemorrhage is increasingly likely as time passes.

292. The answer is a. (*Victor, p 574.*) Infants with this defect in development of the myenteric plexus are susceptible to intestinal obstruction and megacolon development. The affected infants are often misconstrued as merely colicky shortly after birth, but recurrent bouts of constipation, diarrhea, and vomiting point to more serious disturbances of intestinal motility. Intestinal obstruction is likely to become complete within the first year of life and may be fatal if not surgically corrected. The failure of migration of neural crest cells has been linked to a defect on chromosome 10.

293. The answer is b. (*Lee, pp 143–148.*) In the tomogram, the first cervical vertebra, or atlas, is incompletely formed. The most ventral elements are apparent to the left of the left-pointing arrowhead, but the cortical bone of these elements is continuous with that of the skull. The elements of C1 that have formed have simply fused to the base of the skull. This assimilation of the atlas to the base of the skull is a congenital abnormality. It is often associated with a Chiari malformation of the hindbrain.

294. The answer is e. (*Lee, pp 143–148.*) This abnormally situated axis (C2) qualifies as basilar invagination of the skull. If the medulla oblongata is situated at a normal level, it is at risk of compression, but posterior fossa contents may be so caudally displaced that pontine structures are also at risk of compression. Hydrocephalus may develop with this degree of basilar invagination by virtue of obstruction of the flow of CSF through the foramen magnum. Syringomyelia or syringobulbia are occasionally associated with this anatomic variant, but they probably develop as a consequence of cervical cord or brainstem damage.

295. The answer is b. (*Victor, p 1067.*) Men with the fragile X syndrome have hyperextensible joints and prominent thumbs, but carrier women may appear quite normal. The abnormal chromosome may be detected in fetal lymphocytes and fibroblasts, thereby allowing for prenatal screening. Epilepsy develops in many affected persons, but the seizures are usually easily controlled, unlike the case with other hereditary causes of epilepsy.

296. The answer is e. (*Victor, pp 1008–1009.*) Phenylketonuria is inherited as an autosomal recessive trait. It occurs in at least two forms. In one form, intolerance of phenylalanine is extreme, and dietary intake of that amino acid must be restricted from birth. Alternatively, some persons have hyperphenylalaninemia without PKU. This latter group does not have the CNS damage seen with in utero exposure to high phenylalanine levels. Such in utero exposure will occur if the mother is homozygous for PKU. If the mother is normal, infants with PKU are born with essentially normal nervous systems. Damage develops after birth in the susceptible group as serum phenylalanine levels rise.

297. The answer is b. (*Bradley p 2334.*) Sulfatide granules may be evident in nerve tissue, as well as in tissue outside the nervous system, in persons with metachromatic leukodystrophy. The disease is usually fatal within a few years of obvious symptoms. At autopsy, there may be evidence of dysmyelination or demyelination in the CNS, as well as in the peripheral nervous system.

298. The answer is b. (*Victor, pp 997–998.*) Niemann-Pick disease is inherited as an autosomal recessive trait. By 9 months of age, patients with the infantile form usually have prominent hepatosplenomegaly. A deficiency of sphingomyelinase in hepatocytes is diagnostic for the disease.

299. The answer is b. (*Bradley p 2539.*) To what extent the antiepileptic divalproex sodium increases the risk of defects of neural tube closure, such as meningomyelocele, is debatable, but there is at least some increase in the risk. Many agents have been linked to problems with neural tube formation or closure, but none causes problems in a large segment of the population. Colchicine, papaverine, and caffeine, as well as irradiation, hyperthermia, antimetabolites, and salicylates, may increase the risk of neural tube malformations. The vitamin most clearly implicated in cases involving hypervitaminosis is vitamin A. Congenital malformations as a group are slightly increased in the offspring of women with epilepsy even if they are not taking antiepileptic drugs before or during pregnancy. The importance of folate supplementation in women with a prior history of neural tube defect has been shown in several studies and is the basis of the recommendation for the use of folate supplementation during the first trimester of pregnancy. Agenesis of the corpus callosum is a component of several developmental disorders of the CNS, including Chiari syndromes. Kallmann syndrome is a congenital disturbance of the hypothalamus that results in anosmia, hypogonadism, and other maturational problems that become more evident when puberty fails to occur.

300. The answer is b. (*Greenberg, pp 586–587.*) On coronal sections of the brain, the lateral ventricles will have a typical batwing conformation if the patient has agenesis of the corpus callosum. The third ventricle may be dilated and may open onto the surface of the brain. Patients with this congenital anomaly may be asymptomatic or may exhibit a variety of cognitive disorders. In Aicardi syndrome, agenesis of the corpus callosum is associated with retardation, epilepsy, vertebral anomalies, and chorioretinitis.

301. The answer is d. (*Bradley p 2334.*) Hexosaminidase deficiencies produce Sandhoff's and Tay-Sachs diseases. Glucocerebrosidase is deficient in Gaucher's disease. Phosphofructokinase deficiency is usually symptomatic as a disturbance of skeletal muscle function. The enzymatic defect in metachromatic leukodystrophy is transmitted in an autosomal recessive fashion. The affected person usually has retardation, ataxia, spasticity, and sensory disturbances, but individual elements of this disorder may appear alone in less serious cases. The disease is usually symptomatic during infancy.

302. The answer is b. (*Victor, pp 1009–1010.*) With Hartnup's disease there is intestinal malabsorption of tryptophan and other neutral amino acids. Tryptophan serves as a precursor for nicotinamide, but with more than 400 mg of nicotinamide daily, the tryptophan malabsorption becomes less problematic. Inheritance appears to be autosomal recessive. Affected children develop a scaly erythematous rash on the face similar to that seen with pellagra. The ataxia exhibited may be episodic.

303. The answer is c. (*Bradley, p 80.*) With the fragile X syndrome, the terminal elements of the long arm of the abnormal X chromosome appear stretched or broken away from the rest of the chromosome. Retardation usually becomes evident during childhood. Affected men have large ears, a high-arched palate, hypotelorism, and large testes. Autism also occurs among affected men.

304. The answer is e. (*Bradley pp 1881–1884.*) All of these disturbances will produce intracranial calcifications in some cases. The calcifications in Sturge-Weber syndrome follow the gyral pattern of the cerebral cortex and consequently produce the railroad track pattern that is evident on plain x-ray of the skull. Calcium is deposited in the brain of the patient with

Sturge-Weber syndrome, presumably because the abnormal vessels overlying the brain allow calcium, as well as iron, across the defective blood-brain barrier. Craniopharyngioma and acoustic schwannoma produce calcifications, but these are obviously outside the cerebral cortex.

305. The answer is e. (*Swaiman, pp 539–540.*) This man has signs of cerebellar dysfunction. That the deficit has been slowly progressive and is not associated with cognitive dysfunction makes it especially likely that a structural lesion in the posterior fossa is responsible for the deficit. Because the lesion need not disturb the external shape of the cerebellum, a posterior fossa myelogram will not necessarily yield an answer. The CT scan will show if there is an intraparenchymal or extraparenchymal lesion. Drug abuse is not likely to be a factor in this cerebellar syndrome, because all the phenomena that are observed on examination are coordination problems rather than combined cognitive and motor functions.

306. The answer is c. (*Swaiman, pp 539–540.*) The association of erythrocytosis with cerebellar signs, microscopic hematuria, and hepatosplenomegaly suggests von Hippel-Lindau syndrome. This hereditary disorder is characterized by polycystic liver disease, polycystic kidney disease, retinal angiomas (telangiectasia), and cerebellar tumors. This is an autosomal dominant inherited disorder with variable penetrance. Men are more commonly affected than women. Although neoplastic cysts may develop in the cerebellum in persons with von Hippel-Lindau syndrome, these usually do not become sufficiently large to cause an obstructive hydrocephalus. Other abnormalities that occur with this syndrome include adenomas in many organs. Hemangiomas may be evident in the bones, adrenals, and ovaries. Hemangioblastomas may develop in the spinal cord or brainstem, as well as in the cerebellum. This syndrome is not associated with acoustic schwannomas that could cause bilateral hearing loss, and it is not accompanied by peripheral neuropathy, which could cause diffuse hyporeflexia.

307. The answer is c. (*Bradley p 2336.*) Abetalipoproteinemia (Bassen-Kornzweig syndrome) usually becomes symptomatic during early childhood. The peripheral blood smear will exhibit abnormally shaped erythrocytes (acanthocytes), and the plasma lipid profile will reveal a very low cholesterol and triglyceride content. Acanthocytes are spiked or crenated RBCs. These are an unusual hematologic finding in patients with ataxia and are often diagnostic of abetalipoproteinemia. Autopsy examination of the CNS in patients with abetalipoproteinemia reveals posterior column and spinocerebellar tract degeneration. The initial complaints are similar to the spinocerebellar signs of Friedreich's disease. Position sense is lost and extensor plantar responses develop as the disease progresses. As is true for Friedreich's disease, dementia is not an obvious part of the syndrome. Deficits accumulate over the course of years. Vitamin E supplementation may retard the disease's progression. The differential diagnosis of retinitis pigmentosa is broad, and includes many other conditions besides abetalipoproteinemia: mitochondrial diseases, Bardet-Biedl syndrome, Laurence-Moon syndrome, Friedreich's ataxia, and Refsum's disease. It may also occur alone as a hereditary disorder linked to chromosome 3. It is characterized by a degeneration of all layers of the retina. Because it is a noninflammatory condition, retinitis is actually something of a misnomer.

308. The answer is b. (*Victor, pp 1069–1073.*) Although the inheritance pattern of tuberous sclerosis is autosomal dominant, the penetrance is variable. A severely impaired child may be born to a negligibly affected parent. Despite the consensus that inheritance is autosomal dominant, estimates of spontaneous mutations in affected persons are as high as 70%.

309. The answer is b. (*Greenberg, p 597.*) A maternal infection with mumps or rubella virus may produce aqueductal stenosis and, as a consequence, hydrocephalus. The aqueduct of Sylvius connects the third ventricle to the fourth ventricle. The lateral and third ventricles enlarge as the choroid plexus produces fluid that cannot migrate to the subarachnoid space to be reabsorbed.

310. The answer is d. (*Victor, pp 661–662.*) Congenital hydrocephalus usually requires shunting to avoid progressive enlargement of the head and thinning of the brain mantle. Dolichocephaly and brachycephaly refer to head shapes, the former being a long, narrow head and the latter a broad head. Neither of these is necessarily associated with any abnormality. Holoprosencephaly is a failure in development of the midline division of the brain, which may give rise to a stillborn cyclops. A variety of conditions will produce congenital hydrocephalus, and any condition that produces apparent hydrocephalus at birth may produce mental retardation. Correction of the hydrocephalus at or soon after birth reduces the probability of retardation as a direct effect of the hydrocephalus, but conditions that cause damage to the brain as well as obstruct the flow of CSF may leave the patient retarded. An uncorrected hydrocephalus may not be lethal for many years.

311. The answer is c. (*Victor, pp 1064–1065.*) Spina bifida may be extreme in some of the children affected by the Arnold-Chiari (type 2 Chiari) malformation. A myelomeningocele may be present at the level of the spina bifida. Spinal cord tissues may extend into this mass and lie just under the skin covering the neural tube defect. Children with obvious spinal defects usually have persistent problems with leg movements and bladder and bowel control.

312. The answer is c. (*Victor, pp 1069–1073.*) Adenoma sebaceum occurs in about 90% of patients with tuberous sclerosis. A depigmented lesion, called a *shagreen patch,* occurs in only about 20% of these patients. Adenoma sebaceum usually becomes apparent over the malar eminences of the face between 2 and 5 years of age and may evolve into difficult-to-treat angiofibromas of the skin. In ataxia telangiectasia, facial telangiectasias may develop. Sturge-Weber syndrome is characteristically associated with a port-wine spot over part of the face. Patients with neurofibromatosis often have café au lait spots, but these do not usually occur on the face.

313. The answer is d. (*Swaiman, pp 539–540.*) Von Hippel-Lindau syndrome is associated with a high incidence of renal carcinomas. These malignant renal tumors usually develop years after the cerebellar hemangioblastomas, liver disease, or polycystic renal disease becomes symptomatic. People surviving intracranial hemorrhages caused by the intracerebellar hemangioblastomas often succumb to metastatic renal carcinoma. Treating the intracranial lesions does nothing to reduce the risk of metastatic renal cancer.

314. The answer is a. (*Victor, p 1071.*) Retinal phakomas, which require no treatment, are a principal criterion for making the diagnosis of tuberous sclerosis. Along with adenoma sebaceum and periventricular tubers, they are virtually pathognomonic. Other findings that are typical of tuberous sclerosis include ash-leaf spots, shagreen patches, CNS calcifications, renal tumors, cardiac rhabdomyomas, and seizure disorders.

315. The answer is a. (*Victor, pp 1071–1073.*) By 5 years of age, more than half of patients with tuberous sclerosis will have subependymal glial nodules that have calcified. These nodules usually do not become malignant, but they may enlarge sufficiently to produce an obstructive hydrocephalus. Ventriculoperitoneal shunting may be needed if obstruction develops.

316. The answer is e. *(Greenberg, pp 587–588.)* That the cerebellar elements are not fused in the midline suggests an asymptomatic Dandy-Walker malformation. This congenital disorder of brain formation may become symptomatic soon after birth if an obstructive hydrocephalus develops as one facet of the anomaly. In the absence of an obstructive hydrocephalus, the patient may remain asymptomatic throughout life.

317. The answer is e. *(Victor, p 342.)* Adrenocorticotropic hormone is usually given as a gel intramuscularly to control infantile spasms in children with tuberous sclerosis; 40 to 80 mg is divided into two doses. Treatment continues until the infantile spasms abate or the EEG pattern of hypsarrhythmia resolves. This usually requires 6 to 8 weeks of treatment. The ACTH should not be stopped abruptly.

318. The answer is b. *(Victor, pp 1073–1077.)* Café au lait spots in patients with neurofibromatosis are usually larger than a few centimeters and occur in several locations in individual patients. Some have ragged edges and are called *coast of Maine spots*. They occur with both type 1 and type 2 neurofibromatosis, but are much more common with type 1.

319. The answer is b. *(Swaiman, pp 1164–1169.)* The child with congenital weakness, hypotonia, and muscle atrophy may have Werdnig-Hoffmann disease, a congenital motor neuron disease. This is an especially lethal form of motor neuron disease and may limit the child's life expectancy to weeks or months. A similar pattern of disease that appears in older children is less lethal and is called Kugelberg-Welander disease. These types of motor neuron diseases are also known as *spinal muscular atrophies* (SMAs). Anterior horn cell disease is presumed to be a pivotal feature of diseases in this category.

320. The answer is b. *(Victor, pp 996–997.)* More than 90% of children with Tay-Sachs disease develop cherry red spots on the retina. The red spot at the fovea develops as retinal ganglion cells become distended with glycolipid. There are no ganglion cell bodies overlying the fovea, and so the red color of the vascular choroid is apparent in this region but obscured by more opaque glycolipid-engorged cells over the remainder of the retina.

321. The answer is b. *(Bradley, p 1791.)* A static encephalopathy is one in which brain damage has been arrested but neurologic problems persist. Establishing that the brain lesion is not progressive may require extensive testing. A young child with a static motor disorder is said to have CP. Neurodegenerative diseases with slow or stepwise progressions may appear to be static encephalopathies over the course of months, but prove to be progressive encephalopathies over the course of years. The brain lesion with CP is static, but the deficits associated with CP may evolve as the child matures.

322. The answer is a. *(Victor, p 1067.)* The brain of the patient with Down syndrome (trisomy 21) is typically foreshortened. The gyral pattern is simplified, and the frontal lobes are small. The occipital lobes may be slanted, and the overall shape of the skull is abnormal.

323. The answer is b. *(Lee, pp 163–165.)* In utero damage to the fetal brain may be evident at birth as large cysts in the brain. The presence of one or more of these intracerebral cysts is called *porencephaly*. Some pathologists believe that schizencephaly, a related abnormality in which brain segmentation is abnormal, is caused by similar phenomena, which include incidents such as strokes and viral encephalitides in the fetal brain.

324. The answer is d. *(Swaiman, p 534.)* Of the 65% of patients with tuberous sclerosis who are retarded, half are severely retarded. Seizures are invariably associated with retardation. About 20% of patients with tuberous sclerosis develop the Lennox-Gastaut syndrome, with persistent seizures and significant mental retardation. These children usually have a mixed seizure disorder, whereas those without Lennox-Gastaut syndrome most often have complex partial seizures.

325. The answer is d. *(Victor, pp 1247–1248.)* Alcohol abuse in pregnant women is associated with three major kinds of abnormalities in the developing fetus: intrauterine and postpartum growth retardation, dysmorphic facies in the newborn, and effects on the development of the CNS. The broad range of neurologic and systemic abnormalities observed in children born to alcohol-abusing women is referred to as the *fetal alcohol syndrome.* Alcohol is teratogenic at high doses and may interfere measurably in fetal development with exposure at any dose. Although the mechanism of alcohol's effect on the developing brain is not entirely clear, it appears that alcohol acts primarily to impair neuronal migration. This may result in formation of heterotopias (collections of cortical neurons in abnormal locations), cortical disorganization, and malformations of the cerebellum and brainstem. Mental retardation, learning disabilities, hyperactivity, and microcephaly, not macrocephaly, are the common clinical neurologic consequences of fetal alcohol syndrome. Ischemia and hemorrhagic complications are not part of the syndrome. Holoprosencephaly refers to a failure of the two sides of the frontal cerebrum to separate properly, leading to a fusion of the frontal poles and hippocampi with no interhemispheric fissure.

326. The answer is c. (*Lee, pp 143–148.*) Both type 1 and type 2 Chiari malformations are primarily abnormalities of hindbrain development. With the type 1, or adult, abnormality, the cerebellar tonsils extend below the foramen magnum. Affected persons do not usually become symptomatic until they are adults, and then the symptoms are largely referable to the cerebellum. With the type 2 malformation, cerebellar anatomy is usually much more deranged, and the cerebellar vermis lies well below the foramen magnum. Type 2 malformations most often become symptomatic at birth or during infancy and may produce hydrocephalus with retardation.

327. The answer is a. (*Victor, p 1071.*) Microaneurysms and hypervascularity are typically seen with diabetic retinopathy rather than developmental disease. Hemorrhages in the retina would be more typical of hypertensive encephalopathy or a coagulopathy. Neurologic problems that develop in the infant with a prenatal CMV infection include retardation, microcephaly, seizures, and hearing deficits. The virus often causes chorioretinitis, optic atrophy, and architectural changes throughout the brain.

Neuromuscular Disorders

Questions

DIRECTIONS: Each item below contains a question followed by suggested responses. Select the **one best** response to each question.

328. A 65-year-old man was diagnosed with lung cancer 6 months ago. Over the past 2 months, he has had worsening severe proximal muscle weakness. He is most likely to have which of the following?

a. Dermatomyositis
b. Trichinosis
c. Multiple sclerosis (MS)
d. Progressive multifocal leukoencephalopathy (PML)
e. Myasthenia gravis

329. A 2-year-old male child has recently been diagnosed with muscular dystrophy. The parents are highly educated people, but not in the medical field. They have many specific and detailed questions. Which abnormal gene is responsible for the pathology of Duchenne muscular dystrophy?

a. Glucose-6-phosphatase
b. Hexosaminidase B
c. Myosin
d. Dystrophin
e. Actin

330. A 67-year-old woman has noticed blurry vision and weakness over the past 4 months. Her symptoms are always worse toward the end of the day. She undergoes a neuromuscular evaluation, including electromyography, and the diagnosis of myasthenia gravis is made. Which of the following is the most obvious site of disease in myasthenia gravis?

a. Anterior horn cell
b. Neuromuscular junction
c. Sensory ganglion
d. Parasympathetic ganglia
e. Sympathetic chain

331. A patient with amyotrophic lateral sclerosis develops progressive difficulty breathing. His cough becomes totally ineffective for clearing his airway, and he requires a tracheostomy. Facial muscle weakness and fasciculations are obvious at the time the tracheostomy is performed. Which of the following is the most appropriate treatment for this patient?

a. Atropine sulfate
b. Pyridostigmine
c. Edrophonium
d. Amantadine
e. Chest physical therapy

332. A 28-year-old woman has the clinical diagnosis of myopathy and undergoes a muscle biopsy for diagnosis. The pathology demonstrates an inflammatory muscle disease characterized by noncaseating granulomas. Which of the following may have caused her symptoms?

a. Cysticercosis
b. Tuberculosis
c. Sarcoidosis
d. Schistosomiasis
e. Carcinomatosis

333. A 62-year-old woman has limb discomfort and trouble getting off the toilet. She is unable to climb stairs and has noticed a rash on her face about her eyes. On examination, she is found to have weakness about the hip and shoulder girdle. Not only does she have a purplish-red discoloration of the skin about the eyes, but she also has erythematous discoloration over the finger joints and purplish nodules over the elbows and knees. Which of the following is the most likely diagnosis?

a. Systemic lupus erythematosus
b. Psoriasis
c. Myasthenia gravis
d. Dermatomyositis
e. Rheumatoid arthritis

334. The rash typically associated with dermatomyositis is characterized by which of the following?

a. Adenoma sebaceum
b. Shagreen patches
c. Target-shaped erythematous lesions on the extremities
d. A purplish discoloration around the eyes
e. Telangiectasias

335. A 32-year-old woman has several family members with Duchenne dystrophy. She has genetic testing and is known to be a carrier of the gene. A blood test may exhibit substantial elevations in her serum of which of the following?

a. Ammonia
b. Myoglobin
c. Phosphofructokinase
d. Creatine phosphokinase (CPK)
e. Hexosaminidase

336. Duchenne dystrophy affects approximately what percentage of infants?

a. 1 in 3,000 infants
b. 1 in 3,000 male infants
c. 1 in 30,000 infants
d. 1 in 30,000 male infants
e. 1 in 50,000 infants

337. A 2-year-old male child has recently been diagnosed with muscular dystrophy. The parents are highly educated people, but not in the medical field. They have many specific and detailed questions. For a female child to have Duchenne dystrophy, she must have which of the following?

a. Turner syndrome (XO)
b. Klinefelter syndrome (XXY)
c. Two affected parents
d. An affected father
e. An affected brother

338. The spontaneous mutation rate for the dystrophin gene is presumed to be high for which of the following reasons?
a. Men with Duchenne dystrophy do not reproduce
b. The incidence of Duchenne dystrophy is increasing
c. Numerous birth defects occur in families with Duchenne dystrophy
d. Men may become symptomatic after adolescence
e. Genetic studies of eggs in human ovaries reveal an excess of abnormal dystrophin genes

339. Intellectual function in children with Duchenne dystrophy can usually be characterized as which of the following?
a. Markedly impaired
b. Slightly impaired
c. Normal
d. Slightly better than that of the general population
e. Markedly superior to that of the general population

340. In patients with Duchenne dystrophy, which of the following is true?
a. Pseudohypertrophy routinely does not occur
b. Pseudohypertrophy routinely is limited to the shoulder girdle
c. Pseudohypertrophy routinely is limited to the hip girdle
d. Pseudohypertrophy routinely is limited to the calf muscles
e. Pseudohypertrophy routinely is limited to the thigh muscles

341. A 37-year-old man has difficulty relaxing his grip on his golf club after putting. He also is excessively somnolent. Examination reveals early cataract development, testicular atrophy, and baldness. His family says that he has become increasingly stubborn and hostile over the past 3 years. His electrocardiogram (ECG) reveals a minor conduction defect. An electromyogram (EMG) will probably reveal which of the following?
a. Repetitive discharges with minor stimulation
b. Polyphasic giant action potentials
c. Fasciculations
d. Fibrillations
e. Positive waves

342. A 75-year-old man has malaise and slowly progressive weight loss for the better part of 3 months. Laboratory tests reveal a hematocrit of 32%, an erythrocyte sedimentation rate (ESR) of 97 mm/h, and a white blood cell (WBC) count of 10,700 cells per μL. Serum CPK and thyroxine (T$_4$) levels are normal. Which of the following is the most likely explanation for the patient's complaints?

a. Polymyositis
b. Dermatomyositis
c. Polymyalgia rheumatica
d. Rheumatoid arthritis
e. Hyperthyroid myopathy

343. A 32-year-old man develops weakness in his hands over the course of 3 months. Further questioning reveals that he is also having trouble with swallowing. He occasionally slurs his words and has noticed progressive weakness in his cough over the preceding 4 weeks. The weakness is not substantially worse later in the day. He has no sensory complaints associated with his weakness. Sexual function, bladder and bowel control, hearing, vision, and balance are all alleged to be unchanged. The examining physician discovers marked atrophy of the interosseous muscles of both hands. Deep tendon reflexes are hyperactive in the arms and the legs. Extensor plantar responses are present bilaterally. Rectal sphincter tone is normal. This patient's illness characteristically produces electromyographic changes that include which of the following?

a. Fibrillations
b. Markedly slowed nerve conduction velocities
c. Impaired sensory nerve action potentials
d. H reflexes
e. No abnormalities

344. A biopsy is obtained from a clinically affected muscle in a person with several months of progressive weakness. The pathologist reports that there are numerous abnormally small muscle fibers intermingled with hypertrophied muscle fibers. The normal mosaic of muscle fiber types is disrupted. There is no significant inflammatory infiltrate. This pathologic description is most consistent with which of the following?

a. Disuse atrophy
b. Denervation atrophy
c. Muscular dystrophy
d. Polymyositis
e. Hypoxic damage

345. A 52-year-old left-handed woman says that she has a history of myasthenia gravis. When asked about details of the history she says that she was weak. With further prompting the patient becomes belligerent and says that she does not remember any further details. Which of the following is the most common manifestation of muscle weakness with myasthenia gravis?

a. Diaphragmatic weakness
b. Wristdrop
c. Footdrop
d. Ocular muscle weakness
e. Dysphagia

346. A patient with amyotrophic lateral sclerosis dies within 9 months of his initial evaluation. An autopsy is performed, but only the central nervous system (CNS) can be examined. Examination of the spinal cord would be expected to reveal degeneration of which of the following?

a. Dorsal root ganglia
b. Posterior columns
c. Spinothalamic tracts
d. Corticospinal tracts
e. Spinocerebellar tracts

347. The shortest life expectancy is associated with which clinical sign in amyotrophic lateral sclerosis?

a. Atrophy of the interossei
b. Atrophy of the gastrocnemius
c. Fasciculations in the lumbrical muscles
d. Atrophy of the pectoralis muscles
e. Fasciculations in the tongue

Neuromuscular Disorders

Answers

328. The answer is a. (*Victor, p 1484.*) Dermatomyositis occurs as a para-neoplastic syndrome in about 15% of cases overall. Among those over age 40, the proportion of paraneoplastic cases increases to 40% for women and 66% for men. Tumors underlying dermatomyositis may develop in the lungs, ovaries, gastrointestinal tract, breasts, or other organs, but the CNS is generally not the site of a tumor associated with dermatomyositis. Because of the higher probability of malignancy in adults with dermatomyositis, patients diagnosed with this inflammatory disease should routinely undergo a variety of diagnostic studies, including rectal and breast examinations, periodic screens for occult blood in the stool, and hemograms. Sputum cytologies and chest x-rays, as well as urine cytologic studies, are recommended by some physicians. Both PML and MS are strictly CNS diseases. Trichinosis is a parasitic disease that involves skeletal muscle and may produce substantial weakness, but it is not associated with any tumors.

329. The answer is d. (*Bradley, pp 2469–2470.*) Duchenne dystrophy has been incontrovertibly linked to the gene, located on the X chromosome, that makes dystrophin. The more profound the disturbance of this gene, the earlier the disease becomes symptomatic. The gene for dystrophin has single or multiple deletions in affected children. Women who are probable carriers of the defective gene can be checked for heterozygosity and given genetic counseling. Chorionic villus biopsy at 8 to 9 weeks can determine if a fetus that is at risk for the deletion actually carries it.

330. The answer is b. (*Bradley, pp 2443–2445.*) Myasthenia gravis is a disease—or, more accurately, a collection of diseases—in which autoimmune damage occurs at the neuromuscular junction. The postsynaptic membrane is damaged in myasthenia gravis, and the acetylcholine receptor is the principal site of damage. A relative acetylcholine deficiency develops at the synapse because receptors are blocked or inefficient. Symptoms of myasthenia gravis range from slight ocular motor weakness to ventilatory failure.

331. The answer is e. *(Bradley, pp 2257–2258.)* This patient has a motor neuron disease. Pyridostigmine and edrophonium are useful in the evaluation and management of neuromuscular junction disease (e.g., myasthenia gravis). Amantadine is useful in the management of Parkinson's disease and MS, improving mobility in the former and reducing fatigue in the latter. Atropine might be of some use in this patient if he has excessive pulmonary secretions, but conscientious pulmonary toilet performed by an experienced physical therapist is much more likely to be beneficial.

332. The answer is c. *(Victor, pp 1490–1491.)* Sarcoidosis is a poorly understood inflammatory disease that may cause neuropathy as well as myopathy. Multiple organs are usually involved with sarcoidosis, with hepatic or pulmonary disease often the most consistent finding. The non-caseating granulomas help to distinguish sarcoidosis from tuberculosis, a similar disease with an established infectious basis that usually produces caseating granulomas.

333. The answer is d. *(Victor, pp 1482–1488.)* This woman presents with proximal muscle weakness and pain and a heliotrope rash about her eyes. The term *heliotrope* refers to the lilac color of the periorbital rash characteristic of dermatomyositis. This rash surrounds both eyes and may extend onto the malar eminences, the eyelids, the bridge of the nose, and the forehead. It is usually associated with an erythematous rash across the knuckles and at the base of the nails and may be associated with flat-topped purplish nodules over the elbows and knees. Men with dermatomyositis are at higher than normal risk of having underlying malignancies. Psoriatic arthritis may be associated with reddish discoloration of the knuckles and muscle weakness, but the heliotrope rash would not be expected with this disorder. The age of onset for a psoriatic myopathy is also atypical. Similarly, the patient's rashes are not suggestive of lupus erythematosus, although a myopathy may occur with this connective tissue disease as well.

334. The answer is d. *(Victor, p 1483.)* The violaceous, or purplish, discoloration developing around the eyes is called a heliotrope rash (after the flower that has similar coloring). These patients also have erythema over the knuckles. A target-shaped lesion on the limb suggests Lyme disease. Adenoma sebaceum and shagreen patches are skin changes typical of tuberous sclerosis. Telangiectasias over the malar eminences, conjunctivae, and ears occur with ataxia telangiectasia.

335. The answer is d. *(Bradley, p 2474.)* A high CPK in a woman with male relatives affected by Duchenne dystrophy indicates a high probability that she is a carrier of the abnormal dystrophin gene. A normal CPK, however, does not rule out the possibility that the woman is a carrier of Duchenne dystrophy. Even an asymptomatic carrier of the gene may have abnormalities in limb girdle muscles on biopsy.

336. The answer is b. *(Bradley, p 2469.)* Duchenne muscular dystrophy is a fairly common cause of childhood disability, but it is limited to boys. The disease is progressive, but the progression is over the course of years rather than weeks. Affected children rarely survive past adolescence. The incidence of the defect in male fetuses is greater than that in male infants because affected male fetuses have a higher rate of spontaneous abortion than do unaffected male fetuses in families carrying the abnormal gene.

337. The answer is a. *(Bradley, pp 2473–2474.)* Duchenne dystrophy may occur in the person with Turner syndrome if the inherited X chromosome carries the defective dystrophin gene. In the absence of a normal X chromosome, only the defective dystrophin will be produced. The person with Turner syndrome has only one X chromosome but is phenotypically female. Duchenne dystrophy may occur in girls with two X chromosomes if translocations of material from the normal X chromosome inactivate or eliminate the normal dystrophin gene.

338. The answer is a. *(Bradley, pp 2473–2474.)* Despite the drain from the population of males carrying the abnormal gene, the incidence of Duchenne dystrophy is stable. Males often die before they reach sexual maturity or are too impaired after adolescence to mate. There are no changes in the ovaries of women bearing a child with Duchenne dystrophy to suggest that the mutation is arising de novo in the ovary. Women with apparently normal dystrophin genes do, however, give birth to affected sons.

339. The answer is b. *(Bradley, pp 2470–2471.)* Although profound mental retardation is not typical with Duchenne dystrophy, children with the disease characteristically perform more poorly than their unaffected siblings on objective cognitive tests. Persons with the Becker variant, the much milder form of the dystrophy that usually becomes symptomatic during adult life, may have no perceptible cognitive impairments. Women carrying the gene have normal cognitive abilities.

340. The answer is d. *(Bradley, p 2470.)* The calves are usually enlarged in the child with Duchenne dystrophy. Other clinical characteristics include a lordotic posture as weakness evolves in the hip girdle musculature. The gait becomes waddling before the child is unable to walk at all. Affected children invariably exhibit the Gower sign at some time in the evolution of their weakness: the child gets up from the floor by using his hands to walk up his legs and trunk to achieve an upright posture.

341. The answer is a. *(Bradley, p 2485.)* Men with myotonic dystrophy characteristically exhibit problems with relaxing their grip, hypersomnolence, premature baldness, testicular atrophy, and cataracts. The EMG pattern displayed by these patients is often referred to as the *dive bomber pattern* because of the characteristic sound produced when the evoked action potentials are heard. The cardiac defect that evolves in these persons usually requires pacemaker implantation to avoid sudden death. Psychiatric problems also develop in many patients with myotonic dystrophy, but their basis is unknown.

342. The answer is c. *(Victor, p 1572.)* The markedly elevated sedimentation rate, anemia, weight loss, and malaise in a person of this age suggest polymyalgia rheumatica, although the same complaints in someone 20 years younger could not be explained on the basis of this disorder. Fever may also be evident in the affected person. This constellation of symptoms also suggests an occult neoplasm or infection, and investigations should be conducted to reduce the likelihood of overlooking one of these diseases. Polymyalgia rheumatica is an arteritis of the elderly and is improbable in someone less than 60 years of age. The normal CPK activity markedly reduces the likelihood that this myalgia is the result of polymyositis or dermatomyositis. The new onset of rheumatoid arthritis at this age is also improbable. A hyperthyroid myopathy in the face of a normal T_4 level is possible on the basis of an elevated T_3 level, but it is also much less likely than polymyalgia rheumatica in this age group.

343. The answer is a. *(Bradley, pp 2246–2247.)* Electromyogram and nerve conduction studies are a way to establish anterior horn cell damage. The conduction times would be normal even with extensive motor neuron disease, but the pattern of spontaneous and evoked muscle potentials would be abnormal.

344. The answer is b. (*Victor, p 1367.*) Groups of muscle fibers are innervated by individual motor neurons. Characteristically, these muscle fibers will exhibit similar properties on histochemical staining with ATPase, phosphorylase, oxidases, and other markers of cellular characteristics. Adjoining groups of muscle fibers in skeletal muscle may have very different histochemical staining characteristics, but they are usually similar in size. With denervation, all the muscle fibers supplied by the damaged neuron or axon will atrophy. These atrophied fibers may recover if they are reinnervated by branches from adjacent neurons that have not been damaged.

345. The answer is d. (*Bradley, p 2441.*) More than 90% of patients with myasthenia gravis have some type of ocular motor weakness. This ranges from ophthalmoplegia to lid ptosis. Patients usually notice the lid weakness or complain of blurred vision as one of the first symptoms. More severe disease includes limb weakness, difficulty with swallowing, and respiratory difficulties. Patients usually report fatigue that increases as the day progresses.

346. The answer is d. (*Bradley, p 2247.*) This patient had amyotrophic lateral sclerosis (ALS). The disease causes loss of anterior horn cells (lower motor neurons) in the spinal cord and motor nuclei of the brainstem, loss of large motor neurons or Betz cells (upper motor neurons) in the frontal cortex, and degeneration of the corticospinal tract. The myelin sheath of the corticospinal tract axons secondarily degenerates. Often, ALS is called motor neuron disease precisely because it so dramatically targets the motor neurons. Damage to the motor system produces wasting, weakness, and spasticity. Signs of brainstem disease (diaphragmatic weakness, facial fasciculations) early in the course of disease indicate that the prognosis for survival beyond 1 year is poor.

347. The answer is e. (*Victor, pp 1154–1155.*) In ALS, early involvement of musculature supplied by the cranial nerves has a much graver prognosis than early limb involvement. This may be a consequence of disturbed swallowing, with recurrent aspiration as a result, or disturbed ventilatory activity. Fasciculations of the tongue develop with deterioration of hypoglossal nuclei.

Toxic Injuries

Questions

DIRECTIONS: Each item below contains a question followed by suggested responses. Select the **one best** response to each question.

348. A 42-year-old man has had 6 to 15 drinks per day for the past 15 years. He is healthy overall, but has difficulty with tandem gait. Which of the following is the most common site of central nervous system (CNS) atrophy associated with chronic alcoholism?

a. The superior vermis
b. Wernicke's area
c. The supraorbital gyrus
d. The angular gyrus
e. The flocculus

349. An 83-year-old man gives a history of being poisoned by "jake" when drinking illicit alcohol as a young man. After doing some research you learn that "jake" is actually triorthocresyl phosphate (TOCP). TOCP is an organophosphate that may cause lethal neurologic complications by which of the following means?

a. Eliciting massive intracerebral edema
b. Causing a severe motor polyneuropathy
c. Producing widespread CNS demyelination
d. Allowing CNS infections secondary to generalized immunosuppression
e. Inducing status epilepticus

350. A 1-year-old child is brought to the emergency room with an acute encephalopathy. It is determined that the etiology is lead intoxication. With severe lead poisoning, very young children may die of brain herniation secondary to which of the following?

a. Subdural hematomas
b. Epidural hematomas
c. Intracerebral hemorrhage
d. Obstructive hydrocephalus
e. Massive brain edema

351. A 30-year-old man takes a can of beer out of his refrigerator at the end of the day and rapidly swallows a mouthful of its contents before he realizes it is not beer. Within a few minutes he develops severe abdominal cramps, blurred vision, twitching, and loss of consciousness. His wife notifies emergency medical personnel that she had placed some roach spray in the beer can for storage and had left it in the refrigerator to deal with roaches that were nesting there. She claims that she forgot to advise her husband of this. Emergency personnel check the insecticide brand and determine that it is an organophosphate. To counteract the cholinesterase-inhibiting activity of the organophosphate poison, the man should receive which of the following?

a. Methacholine
b. Pyridostigmine
c. Physostigmine
d. Edrophonium
e. Atropine

DIRECTIONS: Each group of questions below consists of lettered options followed by a set of numbered items. For each numbered item, select the **one** lettered option with which it is **most** closely associated. Each lettered option may be used once, more than once, or not at all.

Questions 352–357

Choose the toxin that is most likely to produce each clinical picture.

a. Lead
b. Arsenic
c. Manganese
d. Mercury
e. Carbon monoxide
f. Ergot
g. Nitrous oxide

352. A man working in a poorly regulated felt processing plant develops tremors and memory disturbances over the course of months. He seeks medical help when tremors of his tongue and lips became embarrassing and he is injured during a fall. His family notes progressive irritability and depression. On neurologic examination, he has prominent gait ataxia, limb and facial tremors, and decreased pain and temperature sense in his feet.

353. While vacationing in Latin America, a student buys a brightly painted glazed ceramic pitcher. He drinks orange juice from the pitcher every night while studying. Within 4 months of starting this practice, he develops weakness in both wrists. He consults a physician, who finds weakness on dorsiflexion of both hands, unassociated with any sensory deficits. An EMG reveals evidence of a peripheral motor neuropathy.

354. A 45-year-old woman reports to the police her discovery that her husband has added a suspicious material to her food. She has experienced matrimonial problems for several years and has developed progressive fatigue with frequent headache over the prior 3 months. She consulted a physician when she developed recurrent bouts of severe stomach pain and was told by neighbors that she had been talking to herself and attacking invisible assailants. The physician noted that she had an unexplained anemia and white lines running transversely across her fingernails. She also has had problems with her memory, excessive drowsiness, and a sensorimotor neuropathy with absent tendon reflexes. The physician sent a sample of her hair for analysis and found a neurotoxin present.

355. An Eastern European immigrant who recently arrived in the United States is brought to the emergency room after a seizure. He first developed seizures at the age of 30 and never received treatment. Neurologic examination reveals fasciculations and occasional myoclonus. He is ataxic and has absent deep tendon reflexes. A sensory neuropathy is evident in his legs. Ulcers are evident on his fingers and toes. He acknowledges that his diet was very limited before he immigrated to the United States, and states that most of his calories were derived from rye grains.

356. A 38-year-old miner develops a shuffling gait, tremor, and drooling. His speech is difficult to understand and trails off in volume until it is inaudible. He consults a physician because of easy fatigability and frequent falls. Cogwheel rigidity is evident in his arms and legs. His tremor is most evident when his limbs are at rest.

357. A 35-year-old woman is rescued from a burning building. She is comatose on arrival in the ER. Her skin is cyanotic. Computed tomography (CT) scan of her head shows mild cerebral edema. After intensive care in a burn unit, she recovers markedly, but 2 weeks later, she begins to develop dystonic posturing and bradykinesia. A CT scan now shows hypodensities in the globus pallidum bilaterally.

Questions 358–362

Choose the toxic substance most likely to produce each clinical picture.
a. Ciguatoxin
b. Botulinum toxin
c. Saxitoxin
d. Tick paralysis
e. Ionizing radiation
f. Phencyclidine hydrochloride (PCP)
g. Cocaine
h. *Lathyrus sativus*
i. Ammonia

358. A 45-year-old Portuguese immigrant develops abdominal pain in the early evening after eating grouper for lunch. He later develops fatigue, headache, and paresthesias. He reports on examination that a cold tuning fork feels excessively hot to the touch.

359. A 30-year-old refugee from sub-Saharan Africa is malnourished. She has a subacute spastic paraparesis and gait instability. Cognition, sensory, and cerebellar functions are intact.

360. A 5-year-old girl with long hair is hospitalized during August with a rapidly ascending flaccid quadriparesis over 2 days. She had been camping in the woods with her family during the preceding week. She develops neck, eye, and bulbar paralysis over the 8 h after admission, ultimately requiring mechanical ventilation. Spinal fluid protein and cell levels are entirely normal.

361. A 34-year-old schizophrenic man with a history of Hodgkin's disease in remission since treatment 10 years ago presents with a right middle cerebral artery territory stroke. He is found to have bilateral carotid bruits. There is no history of hypertension, diabetes, or hypercholesterolemia. He does smoke cigarettes.

362. A 27-year-old man with idiopathic cardiomyopathy and right heart failure is admitted to the intensive care unit. Over several days his mental status worsens. He is disoriented and inattentive, but able to follow commands. He has prominent asterixis bilaterally. He improves 24 h later after lactulose is administered.

Toxic Injuries

Answers

348. The answer is a. (*Victor, pp 1224–1226.*) The superior vermis of the cerebellum loses Purkinje cells and exhibits atrophy of the molecular layer in alcoholic persons after years or decades of ethanol use. Alcoholic patients may have gait instability and limb ataxia associated with this injury, but the clinical signs are usually fairly mild considering the histologic damage done by ethanol. White matter in the cerebellum is relatively unaffected.

349. The answer is b. (*Victor, pp 1281–1282.*) Triorthocresyl phosphate damages both upper and lower motor neurons. This damage is usually severe and likely to be permanent. Death may occur within a few days of severe exposure. This material is a common constituent of rat poisons, roach powders, and other insecticides. Oral ingestion is usually required for substantial toxicity. The acute symptoms of poisoning reflect the anticholinesterase activity of the poison. This produces headaches, vomiting, abdominal cramps, excessive sweating, wheezing, and twitching.

350. The answer is e. (*Victor, pp 1277–1278.*) Lead poisoning may cause ataxia and tremor in children exposed to relatively low levels. Chronic exposure routinely impairs psychomotor development and may lead to substantial retardation in very young children. Brain edema develops with toxic lead exposure in infancy and may be lethal even with efforts to relieve the intracranial pressure. Children are exposed to lead in many forms in the environment, including lead-based paint chips from old construction and lead-tainted soil in areas with heavy vehicular traffic.

351. The answer is e. (*Victor, pp 1281–1282.*) Methacholine is a cholinergic agent and would be expected to worsen the symptoms exhibited by this man. Pyridostigmine, physostigmine, and edrophonium are all cholinesterase inhibitors used in the evaluation or treatment of myasthenia gravis, and they too would only hasten this man's deterioration. Atropine is usually given in combination with pralidoxime. This man is at most immediate risk of severe bronchospasm and diaphragmatic paralysis with subsequent respiratory arrest. Even if the patient does survive the acute poisoning, he is at risk for a delayed deterioration of the motor system, which may itself prove fatal and which does not respond to atropine treatment.

352. The answer is d. *(Victor, pp 1280–1281.)* The "Mad Hatter" of *Alice in Wonderland* was a familiar site in the nineteenth century. Persons who cured felt (used in the manufacture of hats) with nitrate of mercury often developed pronounced personality changes, tremor, and ataxia. This type of poisoning is now more typically seen in paper, pulp, and electrochemical plants that use phenyl mercury as part of the manufacturing process. Pathologic changes in the CNS are usually prominent in the cerebellum and include extensive damage to the granular cell layer of the cerebellum. The calcarine cortex of the occipital lobe is also especially vulnerable, and damage to this tissue correlates with constriction of the visual fields.

353. The answer is a. *(Victor, pp 1278–1279.)* Decorative paint and glazes manufactured and sold outside the United States may have very high lead levels. Even mildly acidic solutions, such as orange juice, may leach enough lead out of the paint to produce symptoms in persons exposed over a protracted period to fluids contaminated with the lead. Bilateral neuropathies may develop in adults exposed to lead, and the radial nerves are the most common sites of damage. This neuropathy at its most severe will produce wrist and finger drops as well as occasionally very mild sensory abnormalities in the distribution of the radial nerves. Signs associated with the lead neuropathy may include abdominal pain, constipation, anemia, basophilic stippling of erythrocyte precursors, and a linear discoloration along the gingival margin (lead lines). Penicillamine is used as a chelating agent to reduce the body load of lead.

354. The answer is b. *(Victor, p 1279.)* Acute poisoning with arsenic may cause tonic-clonic seizures or a less dramatic encephalopathy. Hemolysis may be substantial and mucosal irritation may be evident. Death may develop with circulatory collapse if the dose of arsenic is substantial enough. The polyneuropathy that develops with chronic poisoning is resistant to treatment with chelating agents such as BAL. If the patient survives the poisoning, peripheral nerve damage resolves over the course of months or years.

355. The answer is f. *(Victor, p 1275.)* This man's history suggests a nutritional disorder rather than poisoning, but his clinical picture is consistent with chronic ergotism. Ergot is a potent vasoconstricting agent derived from the rye fungus, *Claviceps purpurea.* Currently, the contamination of bread with this material is unlikely in developed nations, but it is still a problem in areas with antiquated agricultural techniques. Chronic ergot poisoning is associated with histologic changes in the CNS, which include degeneration of the posterior columns and dorsal roots. A peripheral neuropathy is also evident, but persons at risk for this disorder are also at risk for other nutritional disturbances that may produce neuropathy.

356. The answer is c. *(Victor, pp 1279–1280.)* Manganese inhalation by miners produces a clinical picture similar to that seen with hepatolenticular degeneration (Wilson's disease). Parkinsonism is the most prominent feature, but axial rigidity and dystonia may also develop. Neuronal loss is evident in several areas of the brain, including the globus pallidus, putamen, caudate, hypothalamus, and cerebellum. Treatment with L-dopa is usually less effective with this heavy metal injury than it is with Parkinson's disease. Agents more likely to produce parkinsonism in the general population include phenothiazines, butyrophenones, and metoclopramide. Metoclopramide (Reglan) is used increasingly after gastrointestinal surgery to manage nausea and other signs of gastrointestinal irritability. Although most physicians do ask about exposure to reserpine-like medications or phenothiazines, other drugs that may cause parkinsonism in susceptible persons are sometimes overlooked.

357. The answer is e. *(Victor, p 1180.)* Carbon monoxide (CO) poisoning can be seen in victims of fires, in those who attempt suicide by carbon monoxide inhalation, or in those who are otherwise exposed to the gas in an unventilated setting. Because of its greater affinity for hemoglobin than oxygen, CO reduces oxygen in the blood and leads to prolonged hypoxia and acidosis. Symptoms may range from confusion and headache at carboxyhemoglobin levels of 20% to coma, posturing, and seizures at levels of 50 to 60%. Characteristic of CO poisoning is delayed neurologic deterioration occurring 1 to 3 weeks after the initial event. Typically, this takes the form of an extrapyramidal disorder with Parkinsonian gait and bradykinesia. Imaging may show the classic hypodensities in the globus pallidum bilaterally.

358. The answer is a. *(Bradley, pp 1736–1737.)* Ciguatera food poisoning occurs in the tropics, but may affect parts of the southern coastal United States, including Florida and Hawaii. Many different toxins are produced by dinoflagellates, which are in turn consumed by reef fish. Ciguatoxin is the best known, and it acts on voltage-gated sodium channels, leading to increased permeability to sodium and increased excitability. Symptoms include abdominal discomfort, nausea, vomiting, and diarrhea, followed by neurological symptoms such as paresthesias, headache, fatigue, ataxia, and myalgias. About 80% of patients complain of a peculiar sensory phenomenon of temperature reversal, specifically characterized by a tendency for cold objects to feel uncomfortably hot. Occasionally, cardiovascular symptoms, including hypotension or shock, may occur due to the effects of the toxin on cardiac muscle cells. Intravenous mannitol appears to have some treatment benefit.

359. The answer is h. *(Bradley, pp 1731–1732.)* Lathyrism is a condition characterized by slow or subacute onset of spastic paraparesis in the setting of excessive dietary reliance on the chickling pea (*L. sativus*) or other members of the *Lathyrus* species. The syndrome typically occurs in epidemics in the setting of famine or war, in which people are forced to rely excessively on this legume. The toxin is thought to be β-N-oxalylamino-L-alanine (BOAA), an excitatory neurotransmitter that can induce the disease in primate models. Damage in the CNS is primarily in spinal cord tracts, especially the corticospinal and spinocerebellar tracts. Demyelination is evident in some affected persons in the lateral and posterior columns of the spinal cord.

360. The answer is d. *(Bradley, p 1578.)* This girl has a clinical syndrome not unlike Guillain-Barré syndrome (GBS). The rapidity of progression, however, and the absence of an elevated spinal fluid protein level, make GBS less likely and tick paralysis more likely. Tick paralysis commonly affects young children, particularly those with long hair that may obscure the tick's location. A careful search for the organism—either *Ixodes holocyclus* (Australia) or a *Dermacentor* tick (North America)—is required in cases of rapidly ascending paralysis of unclear etiology. Removal of the tick will produce dramatic improvement within hours. The responsible toxin of the Australian tick, called *holocyclotoxin*, interferes with the presynaptic release of toxin at the neuromuscular junction.

361. The answer is e. (*Victor, pp 728–729.*) Ionizing radiation may cause accelerated atherosclerosis. Patients with Hodgkin's disease undergoing mantle irradiation may present years later with carotid stenosis due to atherosclerosis. Surgical treatment is made more difficult by the radiation, which can cause scarring of the tissues surrounding the vessels, rendering dissection of the vessel more difficult.

362. The answer is i. (*Bradley, pp 1676–1677, 1679.*) In its early stages, hepatic encephalopathy is characterized by a decrease in the level of alertness; irritability or depression; tremor; and asterixis. As it progresses, lethargy, paranoia, bizarre behavior, dysarthria, nystagmus, and pupillary dilatation may occur. There is good evidence that ammonia is an important factor in the development of encephalopathy, though other mechanisms, including disordered amino acids and neurotransmitters—particularly γ-aminobutyric acid (GABA) and benzodiazepine metabolites—and short-chain fatty acids may play a role as well. Lactulose is the most effective agent in the treatment of hepatic encephalopathy. It appears to work by allowing bacteria in the gastrointestinal tract to assimilate ammonia. Hepatologists have recently updated previous recommendations regarding dietary restrictions on protein in patients with hepatic encephalopathy because it has been recognized that protein consumption is necessary to allow for recovery of liver function.

Eye Disease and Visual Disturbances

Questions

DIRECTIONS: Each item below contains a question followed by suggested responses. Select the **one best** response to each question.

363. A patient reports horizontal double vision. When a red glass is placed over her right eye and she is asked to look at a flashlight off to her left, she reports seeing a white light and a red light. The red light appears to her to be more to the left than the white light. Her right pupil is more dilated than her left pupil and responds less briskly to a bright light directed at it than does the left pupil. The cranial nerve injury likely to be responsible for all of these observations is one involving which of the following nerves?

a. The second cranial nerve
b. The third cranial nerve
c. The fourth cranial nerve
d. The sixth cranial nerve
e. None of the above

364. A 15-year-old obese woman has frequent headaches and early papilledema. Brain MRI and lumbar puncture confirm the diagnosis of benign intracranial hypertension. Which of the following is the treatment of choice for pseudotumor cerebri in a young woman?

a. Lumbar puncture
b. Cesarean section
c. Induction of labor
d. Vitamin A supplements
e. Acetazolamide

365. Which of the following is the most common form of retinal degeneration?

a. Serous retinitis
b. Retinitis pigmentosa
c. Confluent drusen
d. Drug-induced retinopathy
e. Paraneoplastic retinal degeneration

366. A newborn child is being examined. During ophthalmologic evaluation, it is noticed that the red reflex is absent. Which of the following could this indicate?

a. Congenital cataracts
b. Chorioretinitis
c. Retinitis pigmentosa
d. Optic atrophy
e. Holoprosencephaly

367. Glaucoma develops in nearly one-third of children with which of the following?

a. Type 1 neurofibromatosis
b. Type 2 neurofibromatosis
c. Sturge-Weber syndrome (encephalotrigeminal angiomatosis)
d. Tuberous sclerosis
e. Arnold-Chiari malformation

368. A 23-year-old HIV-infected woman presents with visual loss. After testing, the diagnosis of retinitis caused by cytomegalovirus (CMV) is made. Which of the following is the most appropriate treatment for this patient?

a. Cytarabine
b. Vidarabine
c. Ribavirin
d. Interferon
e. Ganciclovir

369. A 52-year-old woman is being evaluated for the acute appearance of a large central scotoma. Which of the following most likely preceded her presentation?

a. Pseudotumor cerebri
b. Chronic ethanolism
c. Chlorpromazine ingestion
d. Methyl alcohol intoxication
e. Isoniazid use

370. A 28-year-old man presents with right eye pain and blurry vision developing over 3 days. After examination and further history, a diagnosis of papillitis is made. How can papillitis be distinguished from the papilledema of increased intracranial pressure?

a. Degree of swelling of the optic disc
b. Associated homonymous hemianopsia
c. Characteristic visual loss
d. Associated limitation of eye movement
e. Loss of red reflex

371. A 19-year-old woman with headaches and visual blurring has prominent bulging of both optic nerve heads with obscuration of all margins of both optic discs. Her physician is reluctant to pursue neurologic studies because the patient is 8 months pregnant and had similar symptoms during the last month of another pregnancy. Her physical and neurologic examinations are otherwise unrevealing. If neuroimaging studies were to be performed on this woman, they probably would reveal which of the following?

a. A subfrontal meningioma
b. Intraventricular blood
c. Slitlike ventricles
d. Transtentorial herniation
e. Metastatic breast carcinoma

372. A 36-year-old woman has tunnel vision in which she reports the same size area of perception regardless of how far from the testing screen the examination is performed. This history often indicates which of the following?

a. Retinitis pigmentosa
b. Neurosyphilis
c. Sarcoidosis
d. Chorioretinitis
e. Conversion disorder

373. A young man with multiple sclerosis (MS) exhibits paradoxical dilation of the right pupil when a flashlight is redirected from the left eye into the right eye. Swinging the flashlight back to the left eye produces constriction of the right pupil. Which of the following is the most likely diagnosis?

a. Early cataract formation in the right eye
b. Occipital lobe damage on the left
c. Oscillopsia
d. Hippus
e. Optic atrophy

374. A 23-year-old woman has 2 days of visual loss associated with discomfort in the right eye. She appears otherwise healthy, but her family reports recurrent problems with bladder control over the prior 2 years, which the patient is reluctant to discuss. On neurologic examination, this young woman exhibits dysmetria in her right arm, a plantar extensor response of the left foot, and slurred speech. Which of the following would be the most informative ancillary test?

a. Visual evoked response (VER) testing
b. Sural nerve biopsy
c. Electroencephalography (EEG)
d. Magnetic resonance imaging (MRI)
e. Computed tomography (CT)

375. Injuries to the macula or fovea centralis typically affect vision by producing which of the following?

a. Bitemporal hemianopsia
b. Nyctalopia (night blindness)
c. Scintillating scotomas
d. Mild loss of visual acuity
e. Severe loss of visual acuity

376. A 64-year-old man who has had hypertension for more than 30 years is being examined. The most obvious changes seen during retinal exam would include which of the following?

a. Retinal tears
b. Optic atrophy
c. Segmental narrowing of arterioles
d. Drusen
e. Telangiectasias

377. Routine funduscopic examination of a 52-year-old man reveals small, discrete red dots located in largest numbers in the paracentral region. Such retinal microaneurysms most often occur with which of the following?

a. Sarcoidosis
b. Chronic hypertension
c. Diabetes mellitus
d. Anterior communicating aneurysms
e. Chorioretinitis

378. A 72-year-old woman presents with the acute onset of double vision. The second image disappears if she covers either eye. Which of the following ocular motor nerves is most likely to be impaired in this patient?

a. Oculomotor
b. Trochlear
c. Abducens
d. Ciliary
e. Müller's

379. A 7-year-old girl acutely develops horizontal diplopia that worsens over the course of a few days. Examination reveals that the double vision is exacerbated by leftward gaze. Red glass testing reveals that the "false" image is from the left eye. She is most likely to have which of the following?

a. Pontine glioma
b. Medullary glioma
c. Mesencephalic infarction
d. Pontine infarction
e. Medullary infarction

380. A 6-year-old girl has left facial pain and blurry vision. Careful examination reveals a deficit of the abducens nerve. Which of the following is the most likely etiology?

a. Ischemia
b. Infection
c. Neoplasm
d. Trauma
e. Hemorrhage

381. A 19-year-old man is hit in the face with a lead pipe. The ocular motor muscle most likely to be injured in this case is that innervated by which of the following?

a. Superior division of the third cranial nerve
b. Inferior division of the third cranial nerve
c. Fourth (trochlear) cranial nerve
d. Sixth (abducens) cranial nerve
e. Long ciliary nerve

382. A 17-year-old girl develops a painful vesicular rash around her left eye. This is followed by blurry vision that occurs only when both eyes are open. She is diagnosed with varicella zoster ophthalmicus. Which ocular motor nerve is most likely to be affected?

a. Superior division of the third
b. Inferior division of the third
c. Fourth (trochlear)
d. Sixth (abducens)
e. Long ciliary

383. A 32-year-old woman has an MRI done because of a first seizure. No etiology for the seizure is found, but there is the incidental finding of an aneurysm. The aneurysm is 5 mm and affects the posterior communicating artery. It is very close to the third cranial nerve. The initial sign of pressure on the third nerve is usually which of the following?

a. Impaired adduction
b. Impaired abduction
c. Impaired depression
d. Impaired elevation
e. Impaired pupillary constriction

384. A 58-year-old man with type 2 diabetes presents with the acute onset of double vision. Examination reveals a deficit of the third cranial nerve. A third-nerve palsy associated with diabetes mellitus is usually characterized by which of the following?

a. Poor pupillodilation
b. Poor pupilloconstriction
c. Sparing of pupillary function
d. Inversion of the affected eye
e. Upward deviation of the affected eye

385. A 65-year-old man is having a neurological exam because of tingling in his feet. During the course of the examination, it is noticed that pupillary constriction occurs with attempted adduction of the globe. This suggests which of the following?

a. Mesencephalic infarction
b. Pontine glioma
c. Acute glaucoma
d. Iridocyclitis
e. Aberrant third-nerve regeneration

386. A 35-year-old man with multiple sclerosis presents with blurry vision. Examination reveals that the medial rectus muscle fails to move synchronously with the contralateral lateral rectus muscle on attempted gaze to either size. When each eye is tested individually, medial rectus function is relatively preserved. In addition, prominent nystagmus is present in the abducting eye. Evidence of internuclear ophthalmoplegia (INO) indicates which of the following?

a. A mesencephalic or pontine injury
b. Thalamic hemorrhage
c. Cerebellar dysfunction
d. Cortical injury in the frontal eye fields
e. Medullary infarction

387. Which of the following is the most likely diagnosis in a 30-year-old woman with evidence of bilateral injury to the medial longitudinal fasciculus (MLF)?

a. Progressive supranuclear palsy
b. MS
c. Subacute sclerosing panencephalitis (SSPE)
d. Progressive multifocal leukoencephalopathy (PML)
e. Botulism

388. A 42-year-old man has horizontal nystagmus in primary gaze and while looking to both the left and the right. The only other examination finding is a slight gait ataxia. Which of the following is the most likely cause of this patient's induced nystagmus?

a. Hysteria
b. Drug intoxication
c. Eyestrain
d. Myopia
e. Hypermetropia

389. A child with rapid downward deviation of both eyes followed by slow upward conjugate eye movements probably has which of the following?

a. SSPE
b. MS
c. Pontine glioma
d. Cervicomedullary junction ischemia
e. Cerebral palsy (CP)

390. A 25-year-old male is being evaluated. Rhythmic jerk nystagmus is elicited by having the patient look at a rotating drum with stripes on it. This finding suggests which of the following?

a. Drug toxicity
b. Brainstem ischemia
c. Parinaud syndrome
d. Unilateral parietal lobe damage
e. No pathologic lesion in the brain

391. A 36-year-old man abruptly loses vision in one eye. His retina appears cloudy and grayish yellow with narrowed arterioles. The fovea appears cherry red, and the vessels that are obvious appear to have segmented columns of blood. Which of the following is the most likely diagnosis?

a. Chorioretinitis
b. Occlusion of the central retinal vein
c. Occlusion of the central retinal artery
d. Optic neuritis
e. Tay-Sachs disease

392. A 62-year-old man with hypertension has an episode in which he suddenly loses vision in his left eye. He is outside walking up the street, as he does every day, when suddenly the vision in his left eye goes black. When he closes his right eye, he can barely see at all. Within 2 h, his vision is back to normal. Amaurosis fugax usually arises because of disease in which of the following arteries?

a. Middle cerebral
b. Posterior cerebral
c. Anterior cerebral
d. Internal carotid
e. Anterior choroidal

393. A 5-year-old girl sustains a cut on her face from broken glass. Initially, the injury appears superficial except for a small area of deeper penetration just above the right eyebrow. Within 4 days, the child develops periorbital pain and double vision. The tissues about the eye are erythematous, and the eye appears to bulge slightly. The optic disc is sharp, and no afferent pupillary defect is apparent. Visual acuity in the affected eye is preserved. Which of the following is the most likely diagnosis?

a. Orbital cellulitis
b. Cavernous sinus thrombosis
c. Transverse sinus thrombosis
d. Optic neuritis
e. Diphtheritic polyneuropathy

394. An otherwise healthy young woman has poorly responsive pupils that are dilated. Visual acuity is normal. A careful neurologic examination reveals bilaterally absent Achilles tendon jerks. Which of the following is the most likely diagnosis?

a. A cervical spinal cord tumor
b. A brainstem glioma
c. MS
d. A posterior communicating artery aneurysm
e. Benign tonic pupillary dilatation

395. A 32-year-old man from a rural area of southern Africa was recently brought to the United States by some of his family members who had emigrated previously. His family says that he was diagnosed with syphilis at age 16 and has taken penicillin off and on over the years, but never completed the prescribed course. Assuming that he has neurosyphilis, which of the following is true with regard to the classic pupillary defect most likely to be observed?

a. Completely normal (no defect)
b. Reacts poorly to light but accommodates well
c. Accommodates poorly but reacts well to light
d. Is pinpoint and regular in shape
e. Is fixed and dilated

396. A 60-year-old right-handed man underwent heart transplantation 2 weeks ago for severe ischemic cardiomyopathy. He had an uneventful postoperative course and went home after 1 week. He is now readmitted from an outside hospital where he was admitted with headaches, increasing confusion, and a generalized seizure. He relates that he has had difficulty seeing for several days. On exam, he has a blood pressure of 180/100. His pupils are equal and reactive, but he has difficulty reading and finding objects presented to him. Motor and sensory function are normal. An MRI shows several areas of T2 signal abnormality in the occipital and parietal lobe white matter bilaterally. A diffusion-weighted MRI sequence, sensitive to the changes of acute infarction, is negative. This patient's history, exam, and laboratory findings are most consistent with which of the following diagnoses?

a. Cyclosporine toxicity
b. Steroid psychosis
c. Occipital lobe infarction
d. Ischemic optic neuropathies
e. Retinal detachment

397. A 60-year-old right-handed man presents with visual loss. About 2 weeks before, he began to notice difficulty seeing the television. Within 1 week, he noticed that the inferior field of vision in the right eye was much worse than the top of his vision. Within a few more days, he noticed the bottom of the vision in his left eye worsen as well. This has been painless. He has otherwise felt well, without headaches or cognitive changes. An ophthalmologist saw bilateral papillitis with white exudates of the nasal part of the discs. There is no history of alcohol use, and the patient has stopped smoking since his heart transplant. On examination, he appears well. Blood pressure is 160/80; pulse is 100 and regular. There are no carotid bruits. Pupils are equal and reactive. Visual acuity is 20/400 OU, with central-inferior scotomas (left larger than right). Neurologic exam is otherwise normal. An MRI scan with and without gadolinium contrast agent, including orbital cuts, is negative, as is CSF examination. This patient's history, exam, and laboratory findings are now most consistent with which of the following diagnoses?

a. Cyclosporine toxicity
b. Occipital lobe lymphoma
c. Tobacco-alcohol amblyopia
d. Ischemic optic neuropathies
e. Retinal detachment

398. Three months following an episode of anterior ischemic optic neuropathy a patient's vision is essentially unchanged. He is able to see in his superior fields, but cannot drive. Funduscopic exam at this time is likely to show which of the following?

a. Papilledema
b. Optic disc pallor
c. Retinal exudates
d. Retinal vein enlargement
e. Drusen
f. Absence of venous pulsations
g. Corkscrew vessels
h. Tilted discs

DIRECTIONS: Each group of questions below consists of lettered options followed by a set of numbered items. For each numbered item, select the **one** lettered option with which it is **most** closely associated. Each lettered option may be used once, more than once, or not at all.

Questions 399–403

For each clinical scenario, select the most probable visual field discovered on tangent screen testing as depicted in the figure.

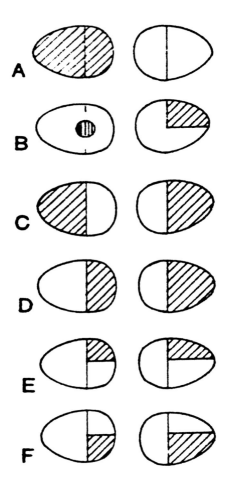

399. A 30-year-old woman with diabetes mellitus and menstrual irregularities complains of chronic headaches with blurring of vision. On examination, she has a lantern jaw, prominent nose, spade-shaped hands, and prominent supraorbital ridges. She is slightly taller than other members of her family.

400. A 17-year-old woman with recurrent enuresis notes pain and visual problems in her left eye. Six months before the development of the visual difficulty, she had transient weakness in both legs for 2 days. Her parents noted slurring and slowing of her speech that appeared to persist long after the transient gait ataxia and leg weakness resolved.

401. A 40-year-old man sustains a gunshot wound to the back of the head. An MRI reveals extensive damage to the left occipital lobe with sparing of the right occipital lobe.

402. A 51-year-old woman has progressive loss of visual acuity in her left eye. Over the course of 5 years, her acuity has deteriorated from 20/20 to 20/400. An MRI of her brain reveals a large meningioma impinging on the left side of the optic chiasm. There is no associated hydrocephalus.

403. A 65-year-old man develops language problems with no loss of consciousness. He is found to have a receptive aphasia, and an MRI scan confirms an area of infarction in the left temporal lobe confined to structures above and lateral to the temporal horn of the lateral ventricle.

Eye Disease and Visual Disturbances

Answers

363. The answer is b. *(Victor, p 285.)* The red glass test produces two images because the eyes are not moving in concert. That the red image appears to the left indicates that the eye covered by the red glass is not moving to the left as much as the other eye. A convenient way to remember this is simply to assume that the eye is not moving where the red image appears to be. This assumes that the red glass is over the impaired eye and that ocular motor function in the other eye is completely normal. Additionally, the outside image is always the false image. That the patient has pain behind the right eye and that the pupil of this eye reacts less vigorously to light than the pupil of the other eye suggests that the right eye is solely (or at least disproportionately) involved. Since the medial rectus and pupillary constrictor are involved, the lesioned nerve must be CN III.

364. The answer is a. *(Victor, pp 667–670.)* With pseudotumor cerebri, removal of some of the CSF produces a protracted lowering of the intracranial pressure. This pressure reduction is desirable because persistent pressure elevations will damage the optic nerve. Pseudotumor cerebri in the pregnant woman usually abates soon after the fetus leaves its mother, but this condition is not serious enough to justify termination or acceleration of a pregnancy. Vitamin excess may cause pseudotumor in some persons. Diuretics are sometimes used to manage patients who are not pregnant, but they are usually less effective than repeated lumbar puncture when that is practical.

365. The answer is b. *(Victor, pp 1165–1166.)* Retinitis pigmentosa is a hereditary degenerative disease involving the retinal receptors and adjacent pigment cells. As this degeneration progresses, small accumulations of pigment appear about the periphery of the retina. Optic disc pallor is evident later in the disease. Retinitis pigmentosa develops along with Bassen-Kornzweig disease (abetalipoproteinemia), Refsum's disease, and other metabolic disorders that produce extensive nervous system damage.

366. The answer is a. (*Victor, p 249. Swaiman, pp 66–67.*) On shining a light through the pupil of the normal newborn, the normal color of the retina is perceived as an orange-red reflection of the light. Failure to perceive that reflection usually indicates opacification of the pathway of light transmission. Several types of intrauterine infections, including rubella and CMV infection, may produce congenital cataracts and impair light transmission in this way. The presence of a distinctive white reflex usually indicates disease behind the lens, such as a scar from retinopathy of prematurity or a retinoblastoma.

367. The answer is c. (*Bradley, p 1881.*) Children with Sturge-Weber syndrome have large port-wine spots on their faces, contralateral hemiparesis, retardation, and seizures, as well as glaucoma. Skull radiographs reveal intracranial calcifications that are associated with leptomeningeal angiomatosis. This syndrome results from a defect on chromosome 3.

368. The answer is e. (*Bradley, p 847.*) All the drugs listed have antiviral activity with effects on CMV in vitro. Ganciclovir is the only one with demonstrable clinical effects on CMV infection. This drug is a 2-deoxyguanosine analogue and has been used for CMV pneumonia and gastroenteritis as well as chorioretinitis.

369. The answer is d. (*Victor, p 264.*) Persons who ingest methyl alcohol will usually be very ill if they survive. Acidosis is a life-threatening complication of exposure to this toxin. Isoniazid, ethambutol, streptomycin, and other drugs may produce similar field cuts, but the blind spots developing with these toxins usually appear subacutely or chronically rather than abruptly.

370. The answer is c. (*Victor, pp 261–262.*) Visual loss is usually substantial with papillitis, an inflammation of the optic nerve head, and inconsequential with papilledema. Patients with papillitis usually also have pain on moving the globe and sensitivity to light pressure on the globe. About 1 in 10 patients have both eyes involved simultaneously. Papillitis is often an early sign of multiple sclerosis.

371. The answer is c. (*Victor, pp 667–670.*) Although papilledema must be considered evidence of a potentially life-threatening intracranial process, optic nerve bulging in this young woman is most likely from pseudotumor cerebri. This is a relatively benign condition that occasionally develops in obese or pregnant women. Cerebrospinal fluid pressure is markedly elevated in these patients, but they are not at risk of herniation. The condition is presumed to arise from hormonal problems. Without treatment, the increased intracranial pressure will produce optic nerve damage with loss of visual acuity.

372. The answer is e. *(Victor, pp 265–266.)* Tunnel vision must be distinguished from concentric constriction. In the latter, the area perceived enlarges as the test screen is moved farther away from the patient, but the overall visual field is always smaller than the normal visual field. Concentric constriction associated with optic atrophy may develop with neurosyphilis. Tunnel vision, on the other hand, is characterized by the patient reporting the same size field even as the test screen is removed farther away. Tunnel vision is not a physiologic pattern of visual loss, and should suggest either conversion disorder or malingering. Significant spiraling of the visual field, in which repeat testing of the same part of the visual field during the same examination leads to a successively smaller field each time, similarly may reflect conversion or malingering, although stress or panic may lead to mild effects of this sort.

373. The answer is e. *(Bradley, pp 730–731.)* The test performed is usually called the *swinging flashlight test,* and the pupillary finding is a Marcus Gunn, or afferent pupillary, defect. It commonly develops in persons with MS as a sequela of optic neuritis. Damage to the optic nerve reduces the light perceived with the affected eye. If the other eye has less or no optic atrophy, the consensual response of the pupil to light perceived by the better eye will constrict the pupil in the atrophic eye, even though direct light to the injured eye does not elicit a strong pupillary constriction.

374. The answer is d. *(Bradley, pp 551–553.)* This young woman almost certainly has MS. Her visual loss can be explained by optic neuritis, and her bladder problems may be due to demyelination of corticospinal tract fibers. Many patients are reluctant to discuss minor problems with bladder, bowel, or sexual function with a physician of the opposite sex. The positive Babinski sign, focal dysmetria, and apparent dysarthria all support the diagnosis of a multifocal CNS lesion. Multiple lesions disseminated in time and space are typical of MS. With MRI, the multifocal areas of demyelination should be apparent. Many more lesions may be evident on MRI than are suggested by the physical examination.

375. The answer is e. *(Victor, p 266.)* The cones of the retina are packed into the macula, and the primary focus of the lens is at the macula. The macula is therefore responsible for visual acuity. Therefore, injury to the macula results in significant loss of acuity, often with preservation of peripheral vision. The macula is usually evident on ophthalmologic examination because it normally reflects a point of light that can be seen through the ophthalmoscope. It is located 3 to 4 mm temporally from the optic disc. Bitemporal hemianopsia is seen in injury to the optic chiasm, as from pituitary tumors. Nyctalopia (night blindness) is seen in retinal degeneration (e.g., retinitis pigmentosa), vitamin A deficiency, and color blindness. Scintillating scotomas are the classic signature of the migraine aura.

376. The answer is c. *(Victor, pp 253–255.)* The vessels apparent on funduscopic examination of the retina are arterioles and venules. In addition to segmental narrowing of arterioles, the retina may exhibit arteriolar straightening and arteriolar-venular compression. The thickened arteriolar wall compresses the venule at the point where they cross, a pattern often referred to as *nicking.*

377. The answer is c. *(Victor, p 255.)* These aneurysms appear as small red dots on the surface of the retina. They may appear as one of the first manifestations of diabetes mellitus and are rarely larger than 90 μm across. They may be more obvious in green light. A proliferative retinopathy may occur along with these microaneurysms in the patient with diabetes mellitus.

378. The answer is c. *(Victor, p 286.)* Injury to the sixth nerve produces a lateral rectus palsy. This type of ocular motor paresis is twice as common as a third-nerve palsy and six times as common as fourth-nerve problems. With lateral rectus weakness, the affected eye will remain inverted on attempts to look straight ahead.

379. The answer is a. *(Victor, pp 286–287.)* An abducens dysfunction with lateral rectus palsy may develop in children with increased intracranial pressure or with direct damage to the brainstem. With a brainstem glioma, both brainstem damage and increased intracranial pressure may develop secondary to the tumor. The adult who develops an acute abducens palsy is also at high risk for tumor. Metastatic lesions from the nasopharynx are especially likely in the adult, but vascular disease is also a significant cause of ocular motor dysfunction in adults, especially in the elderly.

380. The answer is b. *(Victor, p 286.)* Gradenigo syndrome arises with an osteomyelitis of the petrous pyramid. The abducens and trigeminal nerves are affected as they pass close to the tip of the petrous bone. Chronic ear infections may extend to the petrous pyramid and produce this syndrome if they are not properly managed.

381. The answer is c. *(Victor, p 287.)* The fourth cranial nerve innervates the superior oblique muscle. Because this muscle extends far anterior in the orbit, it is at high risk of injury with trauma to the orbit or the full face. The third nerve is especially vulnerable to pressure from aneurysms, but it is usually not disturbed with head trauma unless there are local fractures impinging on it. Injury to the fourth nerve with facial trauma will usually induce a slight head tilt to compensate for impaired intorsion of the affected eye.

382. The answer is c. *(Victor, p 287.)* Varicella zoster, previously known as herpes zoster, spreads to the face along the trigeminal nerve. The fourth nerve is presumably involved because it shares its nerve sheath with the ophthalmic division of the trigeminal nerve. The third and sixth nerves may also be involved with varicella zoster, but this occurs much less frequently than involvement of the fourth nerve.

383. The answer is e. *(Victor, pp 282–299.)* The pupilloconstrictor fibers of the third nerve lie superficially on the nerve. Lesions compressing the nerve impinge on these fibers before they disturb the ocular motor fibers. The third nerve is not involved in abduction of the globe; this is accomplished by the abducens nerve, which controls the lateral rectus muscle.

384. The answer is c. *(Victor, p 287.)* The vessel usually obstructed with diabetic third-nerve injury is deep in the third nerve. The superficial fibers to the iris are supplied by a separate set of vessels, and these are usually spared with diabetes mellitus. With the damaged third nerve, the affected person may complain of pain in and about the eye.

385. The answer is e. *(Victor, p 287.)* Oculomotor fibers that have been damaged reversibly may regenerate and connect to the wrong target. This aberrant regeneration is seen most often with lesions that chronically compress the third nerve. Aneurysms, cholesteatomas, and neoplasms should be suspected in the person exhibiting this type of disturbance.

386. The answer is a. (*Victor, pp 274, 289–290.*) In the MLF syndrome, the patient has incomplete adduction ipsilateral to the lesion in the MLF on conjugate lateral gaze. On attempted conjugate lateral gaze away from the side of the lesion, the patient has nystagmus in the abducting eye. The fast component of the nystagmus is directed temporally.

387. The answer is b. (*Victor, p 289.*) Vascular disease may produce bilateral injury to the MLF in the elderly, but it is an unlikely explanation in the young adult. Injury to the MLF in MS is demyelinating. Bilateral MLF syndromes associated with optic atrophy are virtually diagnostic of MS in persons under 40 years of age.

388. The answer is b. (*Victor, p 291.*) Alcohol and barbiturates are the drugs that most often cause nystagmus. A variety of hypnotic and antiepileptic drugs are also often implicated because they are widely used by the general population. Although the severity of nystagmus in the two eyes may be unequal, it is invariably worse in the horizontal plane of gaze when the nystagmus is an adverse effect of drug use.

389. The answer is c. (*Victor, p 292.*) The phenomenon described is commonly referred to as *ocular bobbing.* It is an involuntary movement that usually develops with pontine damage. Damage to the cerebellum occasionally produces a similar disturbance of eye movements.

390. The answer is e. (*Victor, pp 291–292.*) This type of nystagmus is called *optokinetic nystagmus.* It is a pattern of eye movements that should be elicitable with the normal patient. If the nystagmus is less obvious on rotating the drum in a given direction, the patient may have a parietal lesion responsible for the asymmetric response.

391. The answer is c. (*Victor, pp 255–256.*) Occlusion of the central retinal artery may be due to atheromatous particles, fibrin-platelet emboli, or local retinal artery compression. The visual loss is usually painless and irreversible. Occlusion of the internal carotid artery—the artery from which the ophthalmic and ultimately the retinal arteries originate—need not produce ischemic damage to the retina if collateral supply to the retinal artery is sufficient.

392. The answer is d. *(Victor, pp 834, 860.)* Emboli that arise in or travel through the internal carotid artery may exit to the ophthalmic artery and cause obstruction. The transient ischemia that occurs before the embolus breaks up usually produces transient visual loss in the ipsilateral eye. Amaurosis fugax is by definition a fleeting loss of vision.

393. The answer is a. *(Kasper, p 173.)* The fact that vision is preserved excludes optic neuritis and cavernous sinus thrombosis. Optic neuritis will produce pain in the affected eye and may be associated with a normal optic disc, but visual acuity should be deficient and an afferent pupillary defect should be apparent. Cavernous sinus thrombosis usually produces proptosis and pain, but impaired venous drainage from the eye should interfere with acuity, and the retina should appear profoundly disturbed. With a diphtheritic polyneuropathy, an ophthalmoplegia may develop, but this would not be limited to one eye and is not usually associated with facial trauma. Transverse sinus thrombosis may produce cerebrocortical dysfunction or stroke, but ophthalmoplegia would not be a manifestation of this problem.

394. The answer is e. *(Victor, pp 297–298.)* This pupillary abnormality is called *Adie's tonic pupil.* It is usually seen in otherwise healthy young women and may occur in isolation or in association with absent tendon reflexes. Local trauma to the eye should be considered if only one pupil is affected. If both pupils are affected, drug use should be considered. It is probably due to degeneration of the ciliary ganglia. Although the cause is obscure, it may reflect a mild polyneuropathy. In most cases this is a benign phenomenon.

395. The answer is b. *(Victor, p 297.)* The patient with neurosyphilis may develop an Argyll Robertson pupil. The pupil is usually poorly reactive to light, small, and irregular in shape. Both eyes or only one eye may be affected. Although reactivity to light is deficient, pupillary accommodation with changes in distance from the eye is usually good. The pupillary reaction may, however, be complicated by optic atrophy, which also may develop as a consequence of neurosyphilis. Pinpoint pupils are seen in pontine disease due to interruption of the pupillodilator pathways in the brainstem. The fixed and dilated pupil is generally a sign of third-nerve injury due to compression of the nerve by a vascular or other mass. In the patient with diminished consciousness and contralateral hemiparesis, the concern is for herniation. Other, more benign causes of the fixed and dilated pupil include uveitis, Adie's tonic pupil, and drug-induced irido-plegia (i.e., paralysis of the iris by intentional or accidental application of sympathomimetic or anticholinergic medications).

396. The answer is a. (*Victor, pp 1285–1286.*) Cyclosporine and tacrolimus (FK 506) may both induce a syndrome resembling hypertensive encephalopathy, which has been called by some *reversible posterior leukoen-cephalopathy*, although it involves more than white matter and may also occur in the anterior frontal regions. In the setting of cyclosporine use, patients may develop headache, visual dysfunction related to occipital lobe dysfunction, confusion, and seizures. Usually there is associated hyperten-sion. The visual loss may include cortical blindness or scotomas. Imaging may show bilateral, more or less symmetrical signal changes in the white matter and occasionally the cortex of the occipital and parietal lobes.

397. The answer is d. (*Victor, pp 262–263.*) Ischemic optic neuropathy, often called *anterior ischemic optic neuropathy* (AION), is the most common cause of acute monocular blindness. This condition presents as sudden, painless loss of vision in one eye. Symptoms may progress over several days, and the visual loss is permanent. The visual field defect is typically an inferior altitudinal defect, with involvement of central vision and a conse-quent loss of acuity. In up to one-third of patients, the opposite eye may become involved soon afterward. Hypertension and diabetes mellitus appear to be risk factors, as for most small-vessel disease. The responsible arterial occlusion is of the posterior ciliary artery, a branch of the oph-thalmic artery, which supplies the optic nerve. Typically, this condition is not associated with carotid artery disease. Giant cell arteritis (temporal arteritis) needs to be excluded, because it can be treated with steroids.

398. The answer is b. (*Victor, pp 262–263.*) At the time of the initial injury to the optic nerve, the nerve may appear swollen on funduscopy. As the swelling resolves, however, the disc typically appears pale. This optic nerve pallor serves as a sign of previous injury, and it may be seen after injury due to either infarction (as in ischemic optic neuropathy) or inflam-mation of the optic nerve (as in MS and optic neuritis).

399. The answer is c. (*Victor, pp 265–267.*) This woman has acromegaly, presumably as a result of a pituitary tumor. The growth hormone–secreting tumor responsible will compress the optic chiasm as it extends superiorly out of the sella turcica. Transsphenoidal resection of the tumor may be feasible if the tumor has not extended too far to the side of the sella turcica. Pressure on the optic chiasm will produce a bitemporal hemianopsia.

400. The answer is a. (*Victor, pp 265–267.*) Multiple sclerosis probably caused the ataxia, paraparesis, and dysarthria evident in this young woman. Her loss of vision is presumably due to optic neuritis. This would typically affect only one eye at a time, but the other eye would eventually be involved. The loss of vision would be for the entire visual field of one eye acutely. As the monocular blindness cleared, the patient would be left with an enlarged blind spot.

401. The answer is d. (*Victor, pp 265–267.*) Damage to the left calcarine cortex of the occipital lobe will produce a right homonymous hemianopsia. This will usually split the field of vision exactly at its point of fixation. In rare instances, macular vision from both eyes is preserved, a phenomenon usually referred to as *macular sparing.*

402. The answer is b. (*Victor, pp 265–267.*) With a lesion impinging on the chiasm from one side, there should be a field cut in the contralateral field of the contralateral eye. The upper quadrant is preferentially affected. The ipsilateral eye may exhibit little more than an enlarged blind spot that impinges on central vision, a pattern called a *centrocecal scotoma.* With more substantial damage to the fibers from the eye ipsilateral to the chiasmatic lesion, the patient may have a left nasal hemianopsia, but this rarely appears.

403. The answer is e. (*Victor, pp 265–267.*) Temporal lobe damage produces a superior homonymous quandrantanopsia if there is damage to the optic radiation from the lateral geniculate. Only the lower fibers in this radiation swing superficially in the temporal lobe, extending in front of the temporal horn of the lateral ventricle before swinging back as Meyer's loop to connections in the occipital lobe. Fibers for the superior visual field are in the lower part of the optic radiation.

Disturbances of Hearing, Balance, Smell, and Taste

Questions

DIRECTIONS: Each item below contains a question followed by suggested responses. Select the **one best** response to each question.

404. An 89-year-old man has noticed that his hearing has gradually worsened with aging. This has probably developed because of which of the following?

a. Calcification of ligaments stabilizing the ossicles
b. Weakness of the tensor tympani
c. Neuronal degeneration
d. Weakness of the stapedius muscle
e. Granulation tissue in the middle ear

405. A 65-year-old diabetic woman has aphasia secondary to a stroke involving the inferior division of the left middle cerebral artery. Her hearing is intact. Which of the following correctly reflects why dominant temporal lobe infarction will not produce complete deafness?

a. There is no temporal lobe representation for hearing
b. Each cochlear nucleus projects to both temporal lobes
c. Deafness results with nondominant hemisphere damage
d. Both thalamic and temporal lobe damage must occur
e. Both brainstem and temporal lobe damage must occur

406. A 72-year-old man is having difficulty hearing. He is being tested with a tuning fork. If he has disease of the middle ear, sound transmitted strictly by air conduction will be perceived as which of the following?

a. Louder than that transmitted by bone conduction
b. Quieter than that transmitted by bone conduction
c. Lower-pitched than that transmitted by bone conduction
d. Higher-pitched than that transmitted by bone conduction
e. Oscillating between high and low pitch

407. A 13-year-old girl has a severe case of mastoiditis. Despite treatment, she develops a fluent aphasia. Her aphasia is most likely the result of extension of the infection into which portion of the brain?

a. Frontal lobe
b. Parietal lobe
c. Temporal lobe
d. Occipital lobe
e. Cerebellum

408. A 19-year-old soldier was very close to an exceptionally loud explosion. If her hearing has been damaged, it is most likely what kind of hearing loss?

a. High-tone sensorineural loss
b. Low-tone sensorineural loss
c. High-tone conductive loss
d. Low-tone conductive loss
e. Central deafness

409. A 79-year-old woman is brushing her teeth when she has an intense sensation that the room is moving as if she were on a ship. Examination and testing reveal a cerebellar stroke. Cerebellar damage may be associated with severe vertigo if the tissue damaged is in the distribution of which of the following arteries?

a. Superior cerebellar artery
b. Posterior inferior cerebellar artery (PICA)
c. Anterior inferior cerebellar artery (AICA)
d. Anterior spinal artery
e. Posterior cerebral artery

410. A 62-year-old man has started getting a haircut every week. Whenever he lays his head back to have his hair washed, he has the sensation of spinning. With vertigo that develops on extreme extension or rotation of the head, the patient probably has insufficiency in which of the following?

a. Left subclavian artery
b. Internal carotid arteries bilaterally
c. Vertebrobasilar system
d. Internal maxillary artery
e. Innominate artery

411. A 45-year-old left-handed man has had recurrent attacks of "dizziness." He describes the sensation of feeling the room spinning. The episodes occur abruptly and usually last for approximately 45 minutes. The dizziness occurs about once per month, but may happen more frequently. There is often accompanying ringing and decreased hearing in one ear. Which of the following most accurately describes the early hearing loss in this disease?

a. Over all frequencies
b. Primarily over high frequencies
c. Primarily over middle frequencies
d. Primarily over low frequencies
e. In virtually no patients

412. A 52-year-old diabetic man on multiple medications develops vertigo. Which of the following medications may cause a toxic labyrinthitis?

a. Promethazine
b. Penicillin
c. Dimenhydrinate
d. Acetylsalicylic acid
e. None of the above

413. A 50-year-old man is being evaluated for tinnitus. It is worse on some days than others. Which of the following should he be told may exacerbate the tinnitus?

a. Alcohol
b. Aspirin
c. Glucose
d. Diazepam
e. Steroids

414. A 26-year-old man has multiple café au lait spots. Which of the following tumors is most likely to occur in this patient?

a. Medulloblastoma
b. Acoustic schwannoma
c. Neurofibroma
d. Ependymoma
e. Meningioma

415. A 30-year-old woman has progressive hearing loss. An MRI reveals bilateral acoustic schwannomas (neuromas). Which of the following is the most likely diagnosis?

a. Type 1 neurofibromatosis (von Recklinghausen's disease)
b. Type 2 neurofibromatosis
c. Meningeal carcinomatosis
d. Multifocal meningiomas
e. Disseminated ependymomas

416. The olfactory cortex in humans is located in which of the following locations?

a. Anterior perforated substance
b. Lateral olfactory gyrus (prepiriform area)
c. Posterior third of the first temporal gyrus
d. Angular gyrus
e. Calcarine cortex

417. The hypogonadism and anosmia of Kallmann syndrome usually attract medical attention during which stage of life?

a. The newborn period
b. Infancy
c. Childhood
d. Adolescence
e. Adult life

418. A 22-year-old woman is involved in a head-on motor vehicle accident. She was not wearing a seat belt, and she received a skull fracture when her head hit the windshield. By what mechanism would this patient develop anosmia?

a. Subarachnoid blood causes pial adhesions on the olfactory nerve
b. Injury to the temporal tip injuries the olfactory cortex
c. Torsion on the brainstem injures trigeminal tracts
d. Shearing forces sever filaments of the receptor cells as they cross the cribriform plate
e. Traction on the chorda tympani damages fibers as they course through the skull

419. A 45-year-old man has noticed over the past 6 months that his sense of smell is not as sensitive as it used to be. On examination he has unilateral anosmia, ipsilateral optic atrophy, and contralateral papilledema. Which of the following is the most likely diagnosis?

a. Pseudotumor cerebri
b. Multiple sclerosis (MS)
c. Olfactory groove meningioma
d. Craniopharyngioma
e. Nasopharyngeal carcinoma

DIRECTIONS: Each group of questions below consists of lettered options followed by a set of numbered items. For each numbered item, select the **one** lettered option with which it is **most** closely associated. Each lettered option may be used once, more than once, or not at all.

Questions 420–423

Choose the condition that best matches the clinical scenario.

a. Ménière's disease
b. Cholesteatoma
c. Vestibular schwannoma
d. Benign positional vertigo (BPV)
e. Aminoglycoside toxicity
f. Salicylate toxicity
g. Vestibular neuronitis
h. Posttraumatic vertigo
i. Vertebral artery occlusion
j. Bilateral vestibular hypofunction
k. Bell's palsy

420. A 60-year-old woman has intermittent dizzy spells during the day. Her symptoms are worse when she turns her head to the left, to the point that she tends to keep her head stiff, looking forward. She becomes particularly dizzy when she lies down in bed at night or turns onto her left side. She occasionally wakes up in the middle of the night feeling dizzy. She had a similar experience 2 years ago, which lasted for 2 weeks and then spontaneously resolved. She has otherwise felt well, and her hearing is normal. On examination, putting her head back and the left ear down elicits a feeling of dizziness and nausea associated with rotatory nystagmus, which lasts for 15 s and then resolves.

421. A 34-year-old investment banker has intermittent episodes of vertigo associated with a feeling of fullness in his right ear. These last for several hours. He has had progressive hearing loss in the right ear. There are no other symptoms. He takes no medications and has no history of head trauma.

422. A 47-year-old woman with a history of orthotopic heart transplantation 6 months ago has had a complicated postoperative course and was readmitted 3 months ago with pneumonia. She was treated with gentamicin, vancomycin, and clindamycin, as well as her usual regimen of immunosuppressant medications, lipid-lowering drugs, and aspirin. Since then, she has had severe but stable disequilibrium, with inability to walk without a cane. There has been no hearing loss or weakness.

423. A 72-year-old man awakens with severe vertigo associated with nausea and vomiting. He is ataxic. Over the next several days, he develops numbness of the left side of his body, dysphagia, and hiccups. On examination he has a left homonymous hemianopsia, left-sided sensory loss, dysmetria with the right hand, and no weakness. He has had intermittent episodes of dizziness for the past month.

Disturbances of Hearing, Balance, Smell, and Taste

Answers

404. The answer is c. (*Victor, pp 301–315.*) Presbycusis is the most common cause of hearing loss in the elderly. High-frequency perception is impaired in this disorder because of sensorineural damage. The neurons most likely affected in this degenerative disorder are the spiral ganglion neurons of the cochlea.

405. The answer is b. (*Victor, pp 301–304.*) Hearing in each ear is represented bilaterally even at the level of the brainstem. Lesions rarely produce sufficient damage in the brainstem to cause unilateral deafness unless they are so massive that the patient is unlikely to be responsive to most stimuli and unlikely to survive. If there is unilateral deafness, the patient should be evaluated to determine whether the hearing loss is conductive or sensorineural.

406. The answer is b. (*Victor, p 306.*) The traditional test for detecting conductive deafness is the Rinne test. The vibrating tuning fork is applied to the mastoid process. When the patient can no longer hear the vibration of the fork, it is taken off the skull and moved to the external auditory meatus. With nerve deafness, acuity may be generally reduced, but perception with air conduction will be superior to that with bone conduction. This will also be true in normal persons. With conductive hearing loss, the sound waves are transmitted more effectively to the cochlea directly through the bones of the skull than through the air and along the pathway that starts at the external auditory meatus.

407. The answer is c. (*Victor, pp 508–509.*) Mastoiditis may extend either supratentorially into the temporal lobe or infratentorially into the cerebellum. Cerebellar involvement is likely to produce ataxia, vertigo, nausea, vomiting, and morning headache. Temporal lobe extension causes a fluent aphasia by damaging Wernicke's area in the superior temporal gyrus. The lesion in either the cerebellum or the temporal lobe is usually an abscess formed by bacteria responsible for the mastoiditis. Surgical removal of the abscess is essential in either location, as progression of the abscess in either the cerebellum or the temporal lobe will be lethal.

408. The answer is a. (*Victor, p 310.*) The principal site of damage with acoustic trauma is the cochlea. Mechanical trauma may produce a high-tone conductive loss by perforating the eardrum. A strictly acoustic insult would not be expected to convey enough energy to the tympanum to disrupt it, but it may convey enough energy to the cochlea to shear off receptor filaments from hair cells.

409. The answer is b. (*Victor, pp 844–845.*) The PICA has both medial and lateral branches. The medial branches supply the brainstem. With occlusion of these, vestibular nuclei in the brainstem are infarcted, and vertigo is common. Even with an occlusion limited to the lateral branches, vertigo is likely. If no brainstem damage occurs, cerebellar flocculonodular lobule injury may induce vertigo.

410. The answer is c. (*Victor, pp 842–844.*) The vertebral arteries ascend through foramens in the transverse processes of the cervical vertebrae. With bony spurs on the vertebrae or with severe atherosclerotic disease in the vertebral arteries, flow through the vertebrobasilar system may be transiently reduced when the head is extended or rotated. Because vertigo may be positional without any associated vascular insufficiency, a diagnosis of vertebrobasilar ischemia should be reached only after other causes, such as cerebellar tumor, have been eliminated.

411. The answer is d. (*Victor, pp 319–321.*) Unlike the deficit of presbycusis, lower tones are most susceptible to impaired perception during the initial phases of Ménière's disease. The severity of the hearing loss typically fluctuates considerably. As fluctuations in the low-tone loss abate, high tones become progressively more involved. The attacks of vertigo associated with Ménière's disease usually abate as hearing loss in the affected ear peaks.

412. The answer is d. (*Victor, p 310.*) Salicylates, as well as alcohol, quinine, and aminoglycoside antibiotics, may produce a toxic labyrinthitis with vertigo as a prominent feature. Vertigo is also a common sequela of head trauma or whiplash injury. Promethazine (Phenergan), dimenhydrinate (Dramamine), and meclizine (Antivert) are all commonly used agents to reduce symptoms of vertigo.

413. The answer is b. (*Bradley, pp 254–255.*) Aspirin may produce tinnitus in persons usually unaffected by this problem. Patients on high doses of aspirin for rheumatoid arthritis are especially susceptible to this drug-induced tinnitus. Those patients with chronic tinnitus from acoustic trauma or Ménière's disease will find their symptoms worsen with aspirin.

414. The answer is c. (*Victor, pp 1073–1077.*) Café au lait spots characteristically occur in both type 1 and type 2 neurofibromatosis. Meningiomas, acoustic schwannomas, and other types of CNS tumors occur with these hereditary disorders, but the neurofibroma is the most common lesion. Type 1 neurofibromatosis develops with a defect on chromosome 17, type 2 with a defect on chromosome 22.

415. The answer is b. (*Victor, p 1076.*) Schwannomas most often occur on the eighth cranial nerve, but they may also develop on the fifth, seventh, ninth, or tenth cranial nerves. With type 2 neurofibromatosis, bilateral tumors are more the rule than the exception. The tumors that develop on the eighth cranial nerve usually develop on the vestibular division of the nerve.

416. The answer is b. (*Victor, pp 238–239.*) The olfactory tract divides into medial and lateral striae. The medial stria sends fibers across the anterior commissure to the opposite hemisphere. The lateral stria terminates in the medial and cortical nuclei of the amygdaloid complex, as well as the prepiriform area. This primary olfactory cortex is in area 34 of Brodmann and is restricted to a small area on the end of the hippocampal gyrus and the uncus. This distribution of fibers makes olfaction unique among the senses in that it does not send fibers through the thalamus.

417. The answer is d. (*Swaiman, pp 1317–1318.*) Development of genitalia and secondary sexual characteristics during puberty and adolescence is usually negligible in boys affected by Kallmann syndrome. The olfactory defect is congenital but may be unsuspected until the hypogonadism becomes apparent. The defects responsible for both the anosmia and hypogonadism are developmental rather than acquired. Until the defect in secondary sexual characteristics becomes apparent, the affected person is usually perceived as normal.

418. The answer is d. (*Victor, p 240.*) Anosmia is most likely to develop with head trauma if the trauma is sufficient to cause a skull fracture. If anosmia does occur in the setting of a skull fracture, it is likely to be permanent. With head trauma that does not cause a fracture, anosmia will persist in about 75% of cases.

419. The answer is c. (*Victor, p 231.*) Ipsilateral optic atrophy and contralateral papilledema in association with an intracranial tumor constitute the Foster-Kennedy syndrome. A meningioma of the olfactory groove may produce this syndrome if it extends posteriorly to involve the ipsilateral optic nerve. Compression on the optic nerve by the tumor produces atrophy and interferes with transmission of the increased intracranial pressure down the optic sheath. The increased intracranial pressure is reflected in the papilledema apparent in the contralateral eye.

420. The answer is d. (*Bradley, pp 236–237.*) Benign positional vertigo commonly affects people in middle age or older. It is characterized by recurrent attacks of rotational vertigo occurring on changes in head position, typically lying down or turning onto the side of the affected ear. The symptoms may persist on standing as well, leaving the patient with a continuous sense of disequilibrium. Provocative maneuvers (Nylan-Barany or Hallpike maneuver) are used to confirm that the patient's complaint is due to a peripheral cause of vestibulopathy rather than a central process affecting the brainstem. In a peripheral vestibulopathy, putting the patient's head in a position hanging at 45° off the end of the examining table, with the head turned to the affected side, will produce rotatory nystagmus with a latency of up to 40 s, a brief duration (generally less than 1 min), and fatigability (a decrease in symptoms and signs with successive maneuvers). The cause of BPV is thought to be related to a calcified piece of otolithic material moving within the posterior semicircular canal. Treatment may include vestibular exercises, in which the patient performs provocative maneuvers at home, or maneuvers designed to free the otolith from the posterior semicircular canal.

421. The answer is a. *(Bradley, p 239.)* Ménière's disease is characterized by repeated brief episodes of fullness in the ear, tinnitus, hearing loss, and severe vertigo. The episodes may last from hours to days. Attacks may be so severe that they cause the patient to fall to the ground due to severe disequilibrium. The cause is generally idiopathic, but is thought to relate to distension of the semicircular canal and an increase in the volume of the endolymphatic fluid. For this reason, the condition has been called *endolymphatic hydrops*. Treatment is generally with salt restriction and diuretics. Surgery with endolymphatic shunts is of unproven value.

422. The answer is e. *(Bradley, pp 237–239.)* Aminoglycoside antibiotics may cause vestibulopathy and ototoxicity. The vestibular end organ is affected by streptomycin and gentamicin; kanamycin, tobramycin, and neomycin tend to have a greater effect on the cochlea. Disequilibrium may progress after exposure. The cause is probably related to the fact that these drugs are concentrated in the endolymphatic fluid, exposing the cochlear hair cells to high levels of the drug. Renal disease may exacerbate the effects of the drugs.

423. The answer is i. *(Victor, pp 842–846.)* This patient has a history of progressive vertigo, ataxia, sensory loss, dysphagia, and hiccups, all symptoms of the lateral medullary syndrome, usually due to distal vertebral artery occlusion. This patient's hemianopsia reflects the probable occurrence of occipital lobe infarction, perhaps related to embolism from the occluded vertebral artery. This could have occurred at the time of the lateral medullary stroke or at an independent time. The preceding history of dizzy episodes is indicative of the importance of a thorough evaluation for the cause of dizziness in the elderly patient, particularly when other symptoms occur as well.

Spinal Cord and Root Disease

Questions

DIRECTIONS: Each item below contains a question followed by suggested responses. Select the **one best** response to each question.

424. A 57-year-old woman began having weakness and trouble walking one year ago. Current exam findings include weak, wasted muscles with spasticity, fasciculations, extensor plantar responses, and hyperreflexia. Which of the following is the most likely diagnosis?

a. Dorsal spinal root disease
b. Ventral spinal root disease
c. Arcuate fasciculus damage
d. Motor neuron disease
e. Purkinje cell damage

425. Which of the following is the most likely cause of the spinal cord abnormality evident on this T1-weighted magnetic resonance image (MRI)?

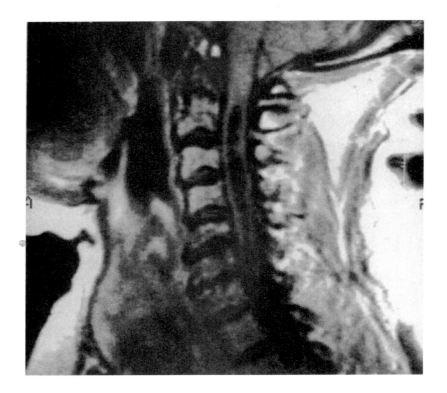

a. Neoplasia
b. Syrinx
c. Infarction
d. Hemorrhage
e. Abscess

426. A 35-year-old woman falls 12 ft off of a ladder and fractures her c-spine, causing damage at the C4 level. She is initially a flaccid quadriplegic with areflexia. This areflexia and flaccidity usually evolve into hyperreflexia and spasticity within which of the following time periods?

a. 2 to 4 months
b. 1 to 2 months
c. 3 days to 3 weeks
d. 1 to 3 h
e. 5 to 25 min

427. After biopsy resection of a lymph node in her neck, a 23-year-old woman notices instability of her shoulder. Neurologic examination reveals winging of the scapula on the side of the surgery. During surgery, she probably suffered damage to which of the following?

a. Deltoid muscle
b. Long thoracic nerve
c. Serratus anterior muscle
d. Suprascapular nerve
e. Axillary nerve

428. A 25-year-old woman is involved in a motor vehicle accident. Among her injuries is a lumbar vertebral body fracture. Which of the following most likely contributed to this injury?

a. Flexion
b. Extension
c. Torsion
d. Spondylolisthesis
e. Subluxation

429. A 35-year-old man injured his thoracic spine in a motor vehicle accident 2 years ago. Initially he had a bilateral spastic paraparesis and urinary urgency, but this has improved. He still has pain and thermal sensation loss on part of his left body and proprioception loss in his right foot. There is still a paralysis of the right lower extremity as well. This patient most likely has which of the following spinal cord conditions?

a. Brown-Séquard (hemisection) syndrome
b. Complete transection
c. Posterior column syndrome
d. Syringomyelic syndrome
e. Tabetic syndrome

430. A 19-year-old man injured his cervical spine in a swimming pool diving accident. Following an initial severe quadraparesis, there was a rapid recovery of much motor function over several weeks. Which of the following would you expect to find in this patient 12 months from now?

a. Fasciculations
b. Fibrillations
c. Flaccid paralysis
d. Hyporeflexia
e. Spastic paralysis

431. The posterior column neurons decussate at what level?

a. At the medulla
b. At the midbrain
c. At the pons
d. At the thalamus
e. Within one or two levels after entering the spinal cord

432. An 82-year-old woman with bilateral leg weakness has a greatly dilated abdominal aorta with a normal thoracic aorta. Which of the following is the most likely cause of this damage?

a. Syphilis
b. Trauma
c. Chronic hypertension
d. Diabetes mellitus
e. Atherosclerosis

433. A 61-year-old man, who smokes five packs of cigarettes per day and has hypertension, had an abdominal aortic aneurysm repair 8 hours ago. The surgery went very well, and there were no reported perioperative complications. Now the patient is unable to move his legs and states that they are "numb." On examination, he has a flaccid paresis of both lower extremities and has impaired pinprick sensation to a T9 level bilaterally. Joint proprioception is normal. Which of the following is the most likely diagnosis in this case?

a. Cerebral stroke
b. Conversion disorder
c. Multiple sclerosis
d. Spinal cord compression
e. Spinal cord infarct

434. The arteria radicularis magna (artery of Adamkiewicz) enters at approximately what level?

a.   C2–C5
b.   C5–C8
c.   T2–T8
d.   T10–L1
e.   L4–S4

435. In a 56-year-old patient with a thoracic spinal cord hemisection, where would you expect the pain and temperature abnormalities to begin?

a.   Exactly at the level of the lesion
b.   Four or five segments above the lesion
c.   Four or five segments below the lesion
d.   One or two segments above the lesion
e.   One or two segments below the lesion

436. The periumbilical area is innervated by which sensory dermatome?

a.   C6
b.   T2
c.   T5
d.   T10
e.   S3

437. Examination of a patient with a cervical syrinx might reveal which of the following abnormalities?

a.   Third-nerve palsy
b.   Calf atrophy
c.   Charcot joints
d.   Atrophy of the intrinsic hand muscles
e.   Grasp reflexes

438. A 36-year-old man is being evaluated for left-hand weakness. On examination, it is readily apparent that he has atrophy of the first dorsal interosseous muscle. This may indicate damage to which of the following spinal roots?

a.   C5 and C6
b.   C6 and C7
c.   C7 and C8
d.   C8 and T1
e.   T1 and T2

439. A 39-year-old woman was involved in a head-on collision at approximately 40 miles per hour. She was wearing her seat belt, but still sustained a cervical cord injury from hyperflexion and extension. A cervical syrinx is most likely to evolve in this patient if there has been which of the following?

a. Intraspinal hyperthermia
b. Intraspinal hypothermia
c. Intraspinal transient ischemia
d. Intraspinal contusion
e. Intraspinal demyelination

440. A 19-year-old man goes swimming in an inland pond in Puerto Rico. Within a few days, he notices itching of his skin over several surfaces of his body. He is unconcerned until several weeks later when he develops lancinating pains extending down his legs and all of his toes. Over the course of just a few days, he develops paraparesis and problems with bladder and bowel control. Within one week, he is unable to stand and has severe urinary retention. Which of the following is the most appropriate plan of action on an emergency basis?

a. Initiate anticoagulation
b. Perform sensory-evoked potential testing
c. Order an MRI scan
d. Place a cervical collar
e. Perform spinal angiography

441. A myelogram is performed upon a patient with a subacute, worsening paraparesis. The cerebrospinal fluid (CSF) and myelogram are both unremarkable except for a slight increase in the CSF protein content. A computed tomography (CT) scan of the spine is unrevealing. Plain films of the spine are completely normal. An MRI of the lumbar cord with gadolinium reveals patchy enhancement at about the L4–L5 spinal cord level. Based on this information, which of the following is the most likely diagnosis?

a. An intraspinal hemorrhage
b. An extraparenchymal meningioma
c. An intraparenchymal ependymoma
d. A transverse myelitis
e. A syringomyelia

442. A 26-year-old recent immigrant from Brazil presents to the hospital with a subacute, worsening paraparesis. The patient had worked in the lumbar industry deep in the Amazon jungle. MRI of the spinal cord is abnormal and a biopsy reveals widespread granulomas. In the midst of one granuloma is an ovoid mass with a spine extending from one side. The pathologist interprets this as a parasitic ovum. If the pathologist is correct, which of the following is the most likely cause of the lesion?

a. *Taenia solium*
b. *Entamoeba histolytica*
c. *Schistosoma mansoni*
d. *Schistosoma japonicum*
e. *Treponema pallidum*

443. A 72-year-old man describes pain about the waist at the level of the umbilicus. The pain is often burning and occasionally shooting. It does not extend down his legs, but he has noticed some weakness in his legs at the time of the pain. With exertion, such as walking, he develops pain in his legs and a tingling sensation in his feet. He has been taking aspirin for the discomfort, but has noticed no substantial change in the sensation. X-rays of his spine reveal no abnormalities. Pain and weakness have become increasingly frequent over the course of several months. Because the man has had urinary hesitancy and frequency in association with an enlarged prostate, he is advised to have a transurethral prostatectomy. A general anesthetic is given for the surgery. On recovering consciousness postoperatively, the man cannot move his legs and has persistent pain at the level of the umbilicus. His plantar responses are bilaterally extensor. Which of the following is the most appropriate emergency evaluation for this patient?

a. Voiding cystometrogram
b. Electroencephalogram (EEG)
c. Somatosensory evoked potentials (SSEPs)
d. Aortogram
e. Penile-brachial index (PBI)

444. The lateral corticospinal tract decussates at what level?

a. At the junction of the medulla and the spinal cord
b. At the junction of the midbrain and the medulla
c. At the junction of the pons and the medulla
d. At the thalamus
e. Within one or two levels after entering the spinal cord

445. Physical examination of a patient who has had a spinal cord infarct reveals preservation of some sensation in the feet. Which of the following would be the most intact modality?

a. Vibration
b. Pain
c. Temperature
d. Two-point discrimination
e. Graphesthesia

446. A 67-year-old man who has smoked heavily for 45 years describes that with exertion, such as walking, he develops pain in his legs and a tingling sensation in his feet. X-rays of his spine reveal no abnormalities. Pain and weakness have become increasingly frequent over the course of several months. The pain and weakness described by the patient with exertion is probably a manifestation of which of the following?

a. Myotonia
b. Myokymia
c. Spinal claudication
d. Spondylolisthesis
e. Spondylolysis

447. A 67-year-old diabetic man underwent repair of an abdominal aortic dissection. The procedure seemed to go well; however, the patient awoke with an upper motor neuron pattern of weakness in both of his lower extremities. Sensation for light touch and joint proprioception were relatively preserved. The CSF analysis associated with this patient's condition is which of the following?

a. An increase in the CSF gamma globulin content
b. A depressed CSF glucose content
c. A protein content of greater than 45 mg/dL
d. More than 100 white blood cells (WBCs) per μL
e. More than 100 red blood cells (RBCs) per μL

448. A patient with a spastic paraparesis has an obvious aortic aneurysm discovered on aortography. The vascular surgeon consulting on the case recommends a bypass procedure. Preoperatively, the patient showed substantial recovery of leg strength and sensation, despite the persistence of bilateral Babinski (plantar extensor) signs. The patient undergoes the surgery and is paraplegic postoperatively with dense loss of sensation of pain and temperature below the level of T10. A follow-up aortogram would be expected to reveal which of the following?

a. Complete occlusion of the bypass graft
b. Complete occlusion of the hypogastric artery
c. Complete occlusion of the aorta below the tenth thoracic vertebra
d. No flow through the artery of Adamkiewicz
e. No flow through the external iliac artery

Spinal Cord and Root Disease

Answers

424. The answer is d. *(Bradley, pp 2246–2254.)* Motor neuron disease in the anterior horns of the spinal cord and damage to the corticospinal tracts or motor neurons contributing axons to the corticospinal tracts would account for these neurologic signs. Damage to the dorsal spinal root would be expected to produce sensory, rather than motor, deficits and would produce areflexia, rather than hyperreflexia, at the level of the injury. Damage to the ventral spinal roots would produce weakness and wasting, but no spasticity or hyperreflexia would develop. Purkinje cell damage would be expected to produce ataxia without substantial weakness. The arcuate fasciculus connects elements of the cerebral cortex not involved in the regulation of strength or motor tone.

425. The answer is b. *(Patten, p 256.)* The sausage-shaped structure in the spinal canal is a syrinx extending from C2 down into the thoracic spinal cord. This is filled with a fluid that appears similar to CSF on MRI. That this patient has syringomyelia independent of neoplasia, infarction, or intraspinal hemorrhage is suggested by the protrusion of cerebellar structures below the foramen magnum. The combination of a low-lying vermis or cerebellar tonsils and syringomyelia points to a Chiari malformation. Although it is inapparent on this MRI scan, the posterior fossa would be expected to be abnormally small and the tentorium cerebelli would insert relatively low on the cranium. Other spinal or spinal cord problems, such as spina bifida and tethered spinal cord, would not be unusual features in association with a Chiari malformation. Even an imperforate anus might be found in the infant with a Chiari malformation, but damage to the cord sufficient to produce paraplegia is most likely with a lumbosacral myelomeningocele. With this lesion, there is a defect in the dorsal aspect of the spinal column with an attendant outpouching of meninges and neural elements from the spinal cord. Potential treatment modalities of syrinxes include laminectomy (to reduce damage to the spinal cord from pressure that develops between the intraspinal cyst and the vertebrae), cyst aspiration, marsupialization (slicing open and leaving open the cyst), and shunting.

426. The answer is c. (*Victor, p 56.*) Spinal shock is a transient phenomenon that occurs with damage to fibers from upper motor neurons. The spasticity that usually develops within a few days of the spinal cord injury is presumed to represent exaggeration of the normal stretch reflexes in the limbs disconnected from upper motor neuron control. The evolution from spinal shock to spasticity is much more typical of spinal cord injuries than it is of cerebrocortical injuries, but even with cerebrocortical injuries there is usually an interval of hours to days during which limbs that eventually become hyperreflexic and spastic are hyporeflexic and flaccid.

427. The answer is b. (*Victor, p 1432.*) Winging of the scapula most often occurs with weakness of the serratus anterior muscle. This is innervated by the long thoracic nerve, whose course starts high enough and runs superficially enough to allow injury to the nerve with deep dissection into the root of the neck. The long thoracic nerve is derived from C5, C6, and C7. Winging is elicited by having the patient push against a wall with the hands at shoulder level. With this maneuver, the scapula with the weak serratus anterior will be pulled away from the back and the vertical margin of the scapula will stick out from the back. Injuries to the long thoracic nerve are usually unilateral and are often due to trauma or surgical manipulation.

428. The answer is a. (*Victor, p 213.*) Extreme flexion of the lumbar spine is likely in automobile accidents and in falls where the person is upright. Fracture of a lumbar vertebral body may be seen in vehicular accidents when the victim is restrained during a high-speed impact by a seat belt without a shoulder harness. The rapid and extreme forward flexion of the lumbar spine may produce a variety of spinal injuries, ranging from fractures to dislocations. Fractures suffered during falls in which the person is upright, such as may occur when someone jumps off a building, are usually compression fractures of the vertebral body. Fracture of the vertebral body will usually produce pain coincidental with the injury. Patients with fractures of the vertebral body that occur without trauma or with inconsequential trauma must be investigated for malignant processes, such as metastatic carcinoma, multiple myeloma, and unsuspected osteomyelitis.

429. The answer is a. (*Victor, p 170.*) Hemisection of the spinal cord results in a contralateral loss of pain and thermal sensation due to spinothalamic damage, and ipsilateral loss of proprioception due to posterior column damage. There is also an ipsilateral motor paralysis due to destruction of the corticospinal and rubrospinal tracts as well as motor neurons. Complete transection of the spinal cord would cause a bilateral spastic paralysis, and there would be no conscious appreciation of any cutaneous or deep sensation in the area below the transection. Posterior column syndrome would result in a bilateral loss of proprioception below the lesion, with relative preservation of pain and temperature sensation. Syringomyelic syndrome results from a lesion of the central gray matter. Pain and temperature fibers that cross at the anterior commissure are affected, which may result in bilateral loss of these sensations over several dermatomes. However, tactile sensation is spared. The most common cause of this type of syndrome is syringomyelia. Trauma, hemorrhage, or tumors are other possible etiologies. If the lesion becomes large enough, then other spinal cord systems become affected as well. Tabetic syndrome results from damage to proprioceptive and other dorsal root fibers. It is classically caused by syphilis. Symptoms include paresthesias, pain, and abnormalities of gait. Vibration sense is most affected.

430. The answer is e. (*Victor, pp 55–58.*) This patient has an upper motor neuron lesion. The damage has been done proximal to the synapse of the anterior horn of the spinal cord. He will therefore develop a spastic paralysis. Fasciculations, fibrillations, flaccid paralysis, and hyporeflexia are all found following lower motor neuron lesions (at the anterior horn cell or more distally).

431. The answer is a. (*Victor, pp 160–162.*) After the primary sensory fiber enters the spinal cord, the ascending branch enters the dorsal columns and travels to the medulla. The fibers from the legs and trunk travel medially in the fasciculus gracilis, while those from the arm and neck travel laterally in the fasciculus cuneatus. These first-order neurons synapse in the medulla, and then the second-order neurons decussate as the internal arcuate fibers and ascend in the medial lemniscus. The second-order fibers synapse in the ventroposterolateral nucleus of the thalamus, which then synapses on the somatosensory cortex.

432. The answer is e. *(Bradley, p 1078.)* Syphilis may produce an aortic aneurysm, but this is characteristically at the level of the thoracic aorta (the arch of the aorta). With aneurysmal dilatation of the aorta, defects in the wall of the vessel may be exacerbated and dissection of the aortic wall may develop. As this dissection extends into branches of the aorta, it usually narrows and may occlude the lumen of the vessels. Diabetes mellitus may contribute to the formation of atherosclerotic damage in the wall of the aorta, but it is the atherosclerosis itself that is most implicated in the eventual deterioration of the vascular wall. Chronic hypertension may develop with damage that involves the renal arteries, but hypertension would not be expected to be the cause of the aortic pathology.

433. The answer is e. *(Victor, pp 171, 1317–1318.)* This patient probably has a spinal cord infarction from an anterior spinal artery occlusion. The posterior cord may be spared, preserving joint proprioception. Bilateral lower extremity deficits without cranial nerve or mental status findings would be an exceedingly unusual cerebral stroke presentation. There is no information, such as psychological stressors or a nonphysiologic exam, to suggest a conversion disorder in this case. Multiple sclerosis causes neurological deficits over space and time. In this case we have a single deficit at a single point in time. History of metastatic cancer or trauma might make the physician suspect spinal cord compression.

434. The answer is d. *(Victor, p 1315.)* The artery of Adamkiewicz is a major anterior radicular artery and may supply the lower two-thirds of the spinal cord. It is at risk of occlusion during abdominal aortic aneurysm repair. Other branches off of the aorta or internal iliac arteries may also supply the thoracic and lumbar cord. The upper segments of the spinal cord are usually supplied off the vertebral arteries.

435. The answer is e. *(Victor, p 170.)* The spinothalamic system is responsible for pain and temperature sensation. It enters the spinal cord through the dorsal root ganglion. The second-order neurons then ascend one or two levels as they cross in the anterior gray commissure. Thus a lesion of the right spinothalamic tract at the T8 spinal cord level would result in a contralateral loss of pain and temperature on the left body beginning at approximately the T9–T10 dermatome.

436. The answer is d. (*Victor, p 160.*) There can be some interindividual variation; however, T10 is clearly the best choice.

437. The answer is d. (*Patten, pp 256–257.*) As the lesion in this region of the spinal cord increases in size, it may affect the lower motor neuron in the anterior horn of the spinal cord, producing weakness in the distribution of the affected motor neurons. Because it is a lower motor neuron lesion, reflexes will be lost rather than increased in the upper extremities, which may at first seem counterintuitive in a spinal cord lesion. The more laterally placed corticospinal tract may be spared, leaving leg function and reflexes relatively normal.

438. The answer is d. (*DeMyer, pp 64–65.*) The first dorsal interosseous muscle is innervated by the ulnar nerve. The fibers of the ulnar nerve reaching this muscle originate at the C8 and T1 roots. If the ulnar nerve itself is the neural element injured, it is usually because of damage at the elbow, where the ulnar nerve runs superficially in the groove over the ulnar condyle. All the interosseous muscles of the hand are supplied by the ulnar nerve: complete transection of that nerve will produce interosseous wasting and impaired finger adduction and abduction. Although the lumbrical muscles are situated alongside the interosseous muscles of the hand, only two lumbricals—those on the ulnar metacarpals—are innervated by the ulnar nerve. The other two lumbricals are innervated by the median nerve. All four lumbricals insert on the extensor sheaths of the fingers and participate in extension of the digits.

439. The answer is d. (*Patten, p 256.*) After cervical cord contusion, cyst formation may occur as damaged tissue is removed. This is especially likely if there has been extensive intraspinal hemorrhage. Ischemic damage may produce similar changes, but the ischemia must be substantial and persistent enough to produce infarction of spinal cord tissue. Demyelination does not lead to syringomyelia, even in cases with extensive intraspinal demyelination.

440. The answer is c. (*Victor, pp 1293–1296.*) A number of spinal cord processes could have produced this evolving paraplegia. Rapid investigation is essential to maximize the likelihood that this young man will recover cord function once the lesion has been treated. Even a reversible lesion left untreated for days or weeks will lead to permanent disability. Magnetic resonance imaging scanning is the best emergent test when available, as it will show compressive lesions as well as processes, such as tumors, inflammation, or infection, that may affect the parenchyma of the spinal cord itself. Vascular lesions, such as spinal cord AVMs, may also be seen on MRI, although spinal angiography is often required to confirm the lesion and guide therapy. Anticoagulation is ill advised, because any one of several processes, such as tumors, vascular malformations, or infections, may have already led to bleeding into the spinal cord or be susceptible to bleeding.

441. The answer is d. *(Victor, pp 1304–1305.)* With an intraspinal hemorrhage, the CT scan would be expected to reveal the clot as a relatively dense mass within the spinal canal. Tumors, such as meningiomas and ependymomas, should have been obvious on MRI if they were producing such dramatic symptoms and signs. Similarly, a syringomyelia should be evident as a cyst that extends over several levels of the spinal cord. With a transverse myelitis, inflammation is largely limited to the substance of the cord, and there need not be an apparent mass effect. This type of reaction may occur with a variety of noninfectious processes, such as MS and sarcoid, or infectious processes, such as viral and parasitic infections.

442. The answer is c. *(Victor, p 1309.)* *T. pallidum* may produce a granulomatous lesion (gumma) in the spinal cord, but this young man has an ovum in the granuloma, which suggests the much more common transverse myelitis attributable to schistosomiasis. Both *S. mansoni* and *S. japonicum* embolize eggs to the CNS, but it is *S. mansoni* that is endemic in Puerto Rico and in locations in South America and that embolizes to the lumbar spinal cord. This patient should be treated with an antischistosomal agent such as praziquantel. Even with treatment, the reversal of disability produced by this spinal cord injury is usually negligible.

443. The answer is d. *(Bradley, pp 1314–1317.)* This patient has symptoms suggestive of ischemic spinal cord disease. The principal source of blood for the spinal cord is the aorta. Vessels that supply the cord are somewhat variable in their origins, but they most commonly arise as branches of the vertebral and hypogastric arteries, as well as of the aorta at the level of the upper and lower thoracic vertebrae. The artery most implicated in a patient with this constellation of symptoms is the great anterior medullary artery (of Adamkiewicz), which arises from the aorta at the level of T10–L1 and supplies the anterior median spinal artery.

444. The answer is a. (*Victor, p 51.*) The lateral corticospinal tract originates primarily in the precentral gyrus (primary motor cortex). These axons then travel in the posterior limb of the internal capsule and then the middle section of the cerebral peduncle. They enter the basal pons and continue as the pyramids in the medulla. At the decussation of the pyramids, the lateral corticospinal tract crosses and then continues down the spinal cord.

445. The answer is a. (*Bradley, p 1315.*) Spinal cord ischemia is usually most severe in the distribution of the anterior spinal artery. The posterior spinal artery is more a plexus of arteries with extensive anastomoses than a discrete pair of blood vessels running along the dorsal aspect of the spinal cord. With a lesion of the spinal cord from ischemia or pressure, the spinothalamic tracts, which are responsible for pain and temperature perception and for providing information for two-point discrimination and graphesthesia, are more vulnerable to injury than are the posterior columns. The posterior columns, which are primarily responsible for vibration and position sense, are supplied by the posterior spinal arteries.

446. The answer is c. (*Bradley, p 1078.*) With exertion, blood that would be available to the spinal cord under resting conditions might be shunted to the more patent blood vessels of the limb muscles. Unlike more typical claudication, in which leg pains develop because of poor blood flow to leg muscles, the leg pains of spinal claudication develop because of shunting of blood to the leg muscles. The pain is a reflection of ischemia to the sensory neurons in the spinal cord. Spondylolisthesis (the slippage of vertebral elements) and spondylolysis (the idiopathic dissolution of vertebral elements) may lead to pain with exertion because of the vertebral instability associated with these commonly linked conditions. However, these diagnoses should be apparent on x-rays. Myotonia and myokymia are disturbances of muscle activity that would not be expected in association with ischemic spinal cord disease.

447. The answer is c. (*Victor, pp 1315–1321.*) With spinal cord infarction, as with cerebral infarction, the CSF is relatively normal. If there is an abnormality, it is most likely to be an elevated CSF protein. The gamma globulin content is not disproportionately increased, as it would be with MS. The cell count of the fluid should be normal. If the RBC content is increased, the physician must suspect hemorrhage into the CNS. An elevated WBC count suggests a wide variety of diseases, including infection, meningeal carcinomatosis, and meningeal lymphomatosis.

448. The answer is d. *(Victor, pp 1315–1321.)* Collateral flow may develop with spinal cord ischemia, but the collateral supply to the anterior cord is likely to fail if the vascular system that supplies the cord is stressed. With the aortic bypass graft, pressure is reduced in the aortic aneurysm and the risks imposed by the dissection in the aortic wall may be reduced, but the pressure forcing blood through the partially obstructed artery of Adamkiewicz is also reduced. With complete failure of flow through this spinal artery, the spinal cord infarction may extend substantially and produce irreversible deficits. Bladder and bowel control is disturbed along with the loss of strength and sensation in the legs.

Peripheral Neuropathy

Questions

DIRECTIONS: Each item below contains a question followed by suggested responses. Select the **one best** response to each question.

449. A 32-year-old man living along the coast of Massachusetts presents with an acutely evolving left facial weakness. Although he has no facial pain or numbness, he does have a diffuse headache. He has no history of diabetes mellitus or other systemic illnesses, but does report newly appearing joint pains and a transient rash on his right leg that cleared spontaneously more than 1 month prior to the appearance of the facial weakness. On examination, he has mild neck stiffness and pain on hip flexion of the extended leg. This man is at highest risk for which of the following causes of a unilateral facial weakness?

a. HIV-associated neuropathy
b. Lyme neuropathy
c. Diphtheritic polyneuropathy
d. Tuberculous meningitis
e. Schwannoma

450. A 62-year-old man is being treated for tuberculous meningitis with isoniazid and rifampin. To avoid additional signs of neuropathy, which of the following agents should be administered along with these antibiotics?

a. Ceftriaxone
b. Thiamine
c. Erythromycin
d. Vitamin B$_{12}$
e. Pyridoxine

451. A patient with a meningitis and facial weakness of unknown etiology had been given isoniazid and rifampin. There was no improvement and she is treated with high-dose steroids. Within 1 week of the introduction of prednisone, she develops pain radiating down the back of her right leg and has difficulty dorsiflexing the right foot. This new symptom most likely represents which of the following disorders?

a. *Borrelia* radiculopathy
b. Diabetic mononeuritis multiplex
c. Isoniazid neuropathy
d. Rifampin toxicity
e. Tuberculous radiculopathy

452. A 12-year-old boy with Lyme disease and bilateral facial weakness is being treated with a cephalosporin. The child's facial strength improves, but he notices twitching of the left corner of his mouth whenever he blinks his eye. This involuntary movement disorder is probably an indication of which of the following?

a. Sarcoidosis
b. Recurrent meningitis
c. Aberrant nerve regeneration
d. Mononeuritis multiplex
e. Cranial nerve amyotrophic lateral sclerosis (ALS)

453. A 25-year-old woman is being examined by her physician. The knee jerk is being tested. The patellar tendon reflex involves sensory fibers of the femoral nerve that originate in which of the following spinal segments?

a. S3–S4
b. S2–S3
c. S1–S2
d. L4–L5
e. L2–L3

454. A 51-year-old factory worker has noticed progressive weakness over the past year. Examination and testing reveal a painless largely motor peripheral neuropathy. Which of the following agents is most likely to be etiologic in this case?

a. Lead
b. Manganese
c. Thallium
d. Cyanide
e. Mercury

455. A 29-year-old woman presents with weakness in several muscles in different limbs. The pattern is lower motor neuron and does not fit with any particular peripheral, plexus, or root localization. Which of the following is the most common cause of mononeuropathy multiplex?

a. Diabetes mellitus
b. Temporal arteritis
c. Sarcoidosis
d. Systemic lupus erythematosus
e. Periarteritis nodosa

456. A very thin elderly woman is having left-sided neck pain. Her family physician attempted to give her a deep intramuscular injection of steroids. She then developed an acute pain radiating down her arm and a subsequent wristdrop. Which of the following is the probable site of injection?

a. Posterior cord of the brachial plexus
b. Medial cord of the brachial plexus
c. Lateral cord of the brachial plexus
d. T1 spinal root
e. C5 spinal root

457. A 17 year-old woman has weakness of left shoulder abduction and elbow flexion, with good strength in hand and forearm muscles. Which of the following is most likely to cause an injury limited to the upper brachial plexus?

a. Node dissections in the axilla
b. Pancoast tumor
c. Birth trauma
d. Dislocation of the head of the humerus
e. Aneurysm of the subclavian artery

458. The most prominent areas of degeneration with Friedreich's disease are in which of the following areas?

a. Cerebellar cortex
b. Inferior olivary nuclei
c. Anterior horns of the spinal cord
d. Spinocerebellar tracts
e. Spinothalamic tracts

459. A 20-year-old ataxic woman with a family history of Friedreich's disease develops polyuria and excessive thirst over the course of a few weeks. She notices that she becomes fatigued easily and has intermittently blurred vision. Which of the following is the most likely explanation for her symptoms?

a. Inappropriate antidiuretic hormone
b. Diabetes mellitus
c. Panhypopituitarism
d. Progressive adrenal insufficiency
e. Hypothyroidism

460. A 27-year-old right-handed man has one week of progressive ascending weakness. Examination confirms a lower motor neuron pattern, and CSF protein is elevated. In retrospect, the weakness was preceded by a severe episode of diarrhea. Which of the following is the most frequent preceding infection before the onset of Guillain-Barré syndrome?

a. HIV
b. Cytomegalovirus (CMV)
c. *Chlamydia psittaci*
d. *Mycoplasma pneumoniae*
e. *Campylobacter jejuni*

461. Friedreich's disease has been consistently linked to a defect on which of the following chromosomes?

a. Chromosome 21
b. Chromosome 9
c. Chromosome 6
d. The Y chromosome
e. The X chromosome

462. A young couple comes to your office because of a family history of Friedreich's ataxia. They are in the process of family planning and have several questions regarding the disease. If a patient with Friedreich's ataxia has children, at what stage of life would a child be expected to become symptomatic if the disease was inherited?

a. Neonatal period
b. Juvenile period
c. Early adulthood
d. Middle age
e. Senescence

463. A 17-year-old male presents with 10 days of progressive tingling paresthesias of the hands and feet followed by evolution of weakness of the legs two evenings before admission. He now has back pain. He has a history of a diarrheal illness 2 weeks prior. On examination, he has moderate leg and mild arm weakness, but respiratory function is normal. There is mild sensory loss in the feet. He is areflexic. Mental status is normal. Spinal fluid analysis in this case is most likely to show which of the following?

a. No abnormalities
b. Elevated protein level
c. Elevated white blood cell (WBC) count
d. Elevated pressure
e. Oligoclonal bands

464. The peripheral neuropathy that would be expected to be seen in a patient with Friedreich's disease develops in part because of degeneration in which of the following?

a. Dorsal root ganglia
b. Spinocerebellar tracts
c. Anterior horn cells
d. Clarke's column
e. Posterior columns

465. A 23-year-old woman develops progressive weakness of the extremities over the course of 1 week. She has further evolution of weakness involving muscles of the arms, face, and respiration. Eventually, she is intubated and placed in the intensive care unit. Nerve conduction and electromyogram (EMG) studies show widespread peripheral demyelination. Therapy with which of the following may help to speed recovery?

a. Corticosteroids
b. Cyclophosphamide
c. Plasma exchange
d. Albumin infusions
e. 3,4-diaminopyridine

DIRECTIONS: Each group of questions below consists of lettered options followed by a set of numbered items. For each numbered item, select the **one** lettered option with which it is **most** closely associated. Each lettered option may be used once, more than once, or not at all.

Questions 466–469

Match each clinical scenario with the most likely diagnosis.

a. Charcot-Marie-Tooth disease
b. Fabry's disease
c. Riley-Day disease (familial dysautonomia)
d. Parsonage-Turner syndrome (brachial plexopathy)
e. Meralgia paresthetica
f. Chronic inflammatory demyelinating polyneuropathy (CIDP)
g. Acute intermittent porphyria
h. Reflex sympathetic dystrophy
i. Leprosy
j. Critical illness neuropathy

466. A 26-year-old woman develops the acute onset of left shoulder pain. Over the following week, she develops weakness in the proximal left arm and mild sensory loss. On examination, she has scapular winging and marked weakness of the left deltoid, biceps, and triceps muscles. The right side is normal, as are her legs. Mild sensory loss in the upper arm is found. She has lost her biceps and triceps reflexes. Her brother recently had a similar problem.

467. A 4-year-old Jewish child has a history of poor sucking at birth, as well as multiple respiratory infections during childhood. He is of short stature and has not been able to eat due to progressive vomiting. On examination, strength is normal, but he is hyporeflexic. There is sensory disassociation, with loss of pain and temperature sensation and preservation of tactile and vibratory sense. The corneas are ulcerated, pupils do not react, and he has orthostatic hypotension.

468. A 56-year-old woman has slowly worsening numbness and paresthesias of the hands and feet, as well as proximal muscle weakness. Bulbar muscles are normal. An EMG shows multifocal conduction block, slowing of nerve conduction, and minimal loss of amplitude of muscle action potentials. Cerebrospinal fluid (CSF) exam shows an elevation in protein to 260, but no increase in the number of cells.

469. A 40-year-old police officer is given pain medications after a femoral fracture. One week later, he presents with confusion, psychosis, abdominal pain, and vomiting. On exam, he is tachycardic, hypertensive, and febrile. He appears delirious. His arms are weak, sensation is relatively preserved, and he is areflexic. His wife relates that he had similar episodes before, when he was in the military.

Questions 470–472

For each clinical scenario, select the most likely condition.

a. Diabetes mellitus
b. Sarcoidosis
c. Thiamine deficiency
d. Pyridoxine deficiency
e. Friedreich's disease
f. Nitrous oxide poisoning
g. Gout
h. Amyloid
i. Abetalipoproteinemia
j. Carcinoma

470. A 49-year-old dentist complains of a pins-and-needles sensation in her feet developing over the course of 3 months. Results of her serum chemistries, blood count, and urinalysis are all normal, but her hematocrit is at the lower limit of normal. She has a positive Lhermitte's sign (electrical pain down the back on flexion of the neck). EMG and NC studies reveal slowed conduction in her sensory nerves. There is no family history of similar problems.

471. A 25-year-old woman with a prior history of visual loss in the left eye and a spastic gait develops impaired pain and temperature perception in her feet. She was diagnosed with multiple sclerosis (MS) shortly after her visual loss. Her left fundus reveals optic atrophy, and her facial movements are asymmetric. Chest x-ray reveals large hilar lymph nodes. Mammogram reveals no apparent carcinoma.

472. A 41-year-old homeless man complains of severe burning in his feet. Vibration, position, pain, and temperature senses are all impaired in both of his lower extremities up to the level of the midcalf. He admits to drinking 1 pt of vodka daily. He was operated on in the past for bleeding from esophageal varices.

Peripheral Neuropathy

Answers

449. The answer is b. (*Victor, pp 768–770.*) The clinical scenario presented is most consistent with a neuropathy of Lyme disease, the infection caused by *Borrelia burgdorferi*. This spirochetal infection is tick-borne and is endemic in the area where this patient lives. The rash on his leg was most likely erythema chronicum migrans, a target-shaped lesion that enlarges as the central area returns to normal. His complaints and examination suggest a chronic meningitis preceded by an arthralgia, a common neurologic scenario with Lyme disease. Facial weakness may be the only neurologic sign of Lyme disease. The neurologic deficits usually appear weeks after the initial rash. Untreated neurologic disease may persist for months. Optic neuritis may also appear in association with the chronic meningitis of Lyme disease. A schwannoma may develop on the seventh cranial nerve, but it would produce unilateral facial weakness followed by signs of brainstem compression. The cranial nerve dysfunctions associated with the early stages of diphtheritic polyneuropathy are a consequence of a toxin released by the infectious agent. Tuberculous meningitis may produce several different cranial nerve deficits. With HIV infection, a peripheral neuropathy may develop, but it typically affects the limb nerves, not the facial nerve.

450. The answer is e. (*Victor, p 1223.*) These antituberculous drugs should be supplemented with pyridoxine to avoid a relative pyridoxine deficiency elicited by the isoniazid. The peripheral neuropathy evoked by the antituberculous agent will appear initially as disturbed sensation in the distal limbs. Paradoxically, pyridoxine overdose may also elicit a peripheral neuropathy, but overdose sufficient to produce a peripheral neuropathy is usually only seen in persons taking many times the recommended daily allowance of pyridoxine in vitamin preparations. It does not develop from eating foods with high levels of pyridoxine. Excessive pyridoxine consumption is usually linked to hypochondriasis or compulsive behavior. Ceftriaxone and erythromycin are appropriate antibiotics in the management of Lyme disease. The cephalosporin is preferred unless the patient is intolerant of that class of antibiotics.

451. The answer is a. (*Victor, pp 1393–1394.*) This patient has, in effect, developed a noncompressive sciatica, or Lyme neuropathy. Dorsiflexion of the foot is controlled primarily by the anterior tibial muscle. The deep peroneal nerve supplies this muscle and arises from the common peroneal nerve just below the knee. A sciatic nerve injury may also produce footdrop, and irritation of spinal roots to the sciatic nerve produces the footdrop that may occur with Lyme radiculopathy. Lyme disease causes painful radiculopathies and peripheral neuropathies. Tuberculosis may cause similar symptoms, but steroid therapy is often useful in suppressing that complaint in chronic tuberculous meningitis. Steroid-induced diabetes mellitus would be unlikely to evolve to the point that a painful neuropathy developed over so short a time.

452. The answer is c. (*Victor, p 287.*) Aberrant regeneration of a cranial nerve is not all that uncommon, but it is more often seen after injury to the third nerve than to the seventh. For unknown reasons, the regenerating motor fibers miss their original targets and innervate new destinations. With cranial ALS, facial twitching occurs, but it is not preceded by unilateral weakness; and it is seen as the weakness evolves, not as it remits. Sarcoidosis may produce facial weakness with aberrant regeneration, but this patient's history does not suggest this idiopathic granulomatous disease. There is nothing to suggest that his Lyme disease is recurring, although recurrent meningitis may develop with inadequate treatment.

453. The answer is e. (*Victor, p 49.*) Myotactic, or tendon stretch, reflexes require intact sensory supplies from the tendons and motor supplies to the muscles involved. The patellar tendon reflex entails contraction of the quadriceps femoris muscle group, a muscle group with four members: the vastus lateralis, vastus medialis, vastus intermedius, and rectus femoris. This reflex requires perception of stretch in the tendon stretch receptors innervated by L2 and L3. With tapping of the tendon that extends from the patella to the head of the tibia, spinal reflex pathways activate contraction of the quadriceps femoris group and evoke extension of the lower leg with straightening of the knee. Damage to the motor supply to the reactive muscles must be profound before the tendon reflex will be lost completely. Corticospinal tract damage will produce hyperreflexia, apparently by disinhibiting spinal cord mechanisms.

454. The answer is a. *(Victor, pp 1393–1394.)* Lead poisoning, especially in adults, produces a painless neuropathy often targeting the radial nerve and resulting in a wristdrop. Lead poisoning in children is likely to produce increased intracranial pressure and cognitive dysfunction. Thallium poisoning may produce hair loss, stupor, gastrointestinal distress, seizures, and headaches, as well as a painful, symmetric, primarily sensory neuropathy. Manganese is also a toxin, but long-term exposure to this metal may produce parkinsonism rather than a sensory neuropathy. Cyanide was long regarded as the cause of an optic neuropathy, but this lethal toxin has probably been unjustly ascribed this capability. Mercury poisoning may produce a sensory neuropathy, but it is generally associated with paresthesias rather than dysesthesias.

455. The answer is a. *(Victor, pp 1396–1399.)* Diabetes mellitus is the most common cause of mononeuropathy multiplex. In this disorder, individual nerves are transiently disabled. The neuropathy usually develops over the course of minutes to days, and the recovery of function may require weeks to months. Various rheumatoid diseases and sarcoidosis produce similar clinical pictures, but temporal arteritis does not typically lead to this type of neuropathy. A vascular lesion is believed to be the most common basis for this type of neuropathy. If the giant cell arteritis seen with temporal arteritis does cause a neuropathy, it is an optic neuropathy with resultant blindness. Unlike the peripheral nerve injuries that develop with mononeuropathy multiplex, this ischemic optic neuropathy of temporal arteritis produces irreversible injury to the affected cranial nerve. The patient who loses vision as part of temporal arteritis does not recover it.

456. The answer is a. *(Victor, p 1428.)* The radial nerve supplies the extensors of the wrist and derives from the posterior cord of the brachial plexus. The brachial plexus arises from C5, C6, C7, C8, and T1. These spinal roots form the trunks of the brachial plexus. C5 and C6 form the upper trunk; C7, the middle trunk; and C8 and T1, the lower trunk. The trunks in turn divide into anterior and posterior divisions, which associate into cords: the anterior division of the upper and middle trunks gives rise to the lateral cord; the posterior divisions of all the trunks give rise to the posterior cord; and the anterior division of the lower trunk gives rise to the medial cord.

457. The answer is c. *(Victor, p 1428.)* The upper brachial plexus includes the fifth and sixth cervical spinal roots. Damage to these roots occurs during a difficult birth if the head and the shoulder are forced widely apart. This could result in stretching or even avulsion of these cervical spinal roots from the spinal cord. Node dissection in the axilla or a Pancoast tumor at the apex of the lung may produce brachial plexus injury, but it is the lower plexus that is vulnerable. Dislocation of the head of the humerus or aneurysm of the subclavian artery will typically injure the cords of the brachial plexus, the final elements of the plexus from which the principal nerves of the arm arise.

458. The answer is d. *(Bradley, p 2173.)* Degeneration occurs primarily in the spinal cord rather than the cerebellum or brainstem in patients with Friedreich's disease. Both the dorsal and ventral spinocerebellar tracts are involved. The other spinal cord structures exhibiting degeneration include the posterior columns and the lateral corticospinal tracts.

459. The answer is b. *(Bradley, p 2173.)* More than 10% of patients with Friedreich's disease develop diabetes mellitus. A more life-threatening complication of this degenerative disease is the disturbance of the cardiac conduction system that often develops. Visual problems occur with the hyperglycemia of uncontrolled diabetes mellitus, but even Friedreich's patients without diabetes develop optic atrophy late in the course of the degenerative disease.

460. The answer is e. *(Victor, pp 1382–1383.)* Serologic studies have shown that *C. jejuni* is the most common infection preceding Guillain-Barré syndrome. Other, less common infections include viral illnesses such as CMV, HIV, and Epstein-Barr virus, Lyme disease, and *M. pneumoniae* infection. Guillain-Barré syndrome has also been associated with surgical procedures, exposure to thrombolytic agents, lymphoma, and certain vaccines.

461. The answer is b. *(Bradley, pp 2173–2174.)* Spinocerebellar atrophy does occur linked to chromosome 6, but this is distinct from Friedreich's ataxia. The site of the mutation responsible for Friedreich's ataxia has been identified on chromosome 9, and the gene product, the protein frataxin, has been identified. Friedreich's disease is inherited as an autosomal recessive defect.

462. The answer is b. (*Bradley, pp 2173–2174.*) Congenital abnormalities are rarely evident with Friedreich's disease, but kyphoscoliosis, pes cavus, and other musculoskeletal abnormalities may become evident quite early in childhood. Gait difficulty usually develops during childhood in persons with Friedreich's disease. Visual loss, syncope, vertigo, and dysarthria may develop during the course of this degenerative disease, but the appearance of these other problems may be decades after that of the gait ataxia. Visual loss may develop with optic atrophy or retinitis pigmentosa. Strictly cerebellar or spinocerebellar tract signs include limb ataxia, nystagmus, dysarthria, and gait difficulty. Systemic problems often found in persons with Friedreich's disease include diabetes mellitus and cardiac conduction defects.

463. The answer is b. (*Victor, p 1382.*) This patient's clinical course is consistent with a diagnosis of AIDP, also known as Guillain-Barré syndrome. Cerebrospinal fluid is typically under normal pressure in this syndrome, and contains no cells in up to 90% of patients. In 10% of patients, 10 to 50 WBCs, mostly lymphocytes, may appear. Protein levels are generally elevated, sometimes to extremely high levels, reflecting the degree of inflammatory activity taking place at the level of the spinal roots.

464. The answer is a. (*Bradley, p 2173.*) Degenerative changes in the peripheral nerves of patients with Friedreich's disease have several bases. Loss of cells in the dorsal root ganglia makes a major contribution to this phenomenon. Additional sites of degeneration that affect the sensory system include the substantia gelatinosa (Lissauer's tract) of the posterior horn and the dorsal roots themselves. The peripheral neuropathy is responsible for the hyporeflexia that is invariably found in the legs of affected persons.

465. The answer is c. (*Victor, pp 1385–1386.*) Treatment of Guillain-Barré syndrome is complicated and is best accomplished in an experienced center. Specific therapies include plasma exchange and intravenous immunoglobulin, which appear to be equivalent in several recent studies. When instituted early (within 2 weeks of symptom onset), these modalities can reduce the period of hospitalization, the length of time on mechanical ventilation, and the time to begin walking again. Corticosteroids do not appear to be of benefit. The role of other immunosuppressants, such as cyclophosphamide, has not been evaluated. 3,4-diaminopyridine is used in the treatment of Lambert-Eaton myasthenic syndrome.

466. The answer is d. (*Victor, pp 1427–1428.*) Parsonage-Turner syndrome refers to an acute brachial plexopathy. It may also be called brachial neuritis or neuralgic amyotrophy. Usually it begins with acute onset of pain in the neck, shoulder, or upper arm. This is followed 3 to 10 days later by the rapid evolution of weakness affecting the proximal muscles of the arm; rarely, the hand or the respiratory muscles may also be affected. Sensory loss also occurs. Some cases are bilateral. Usually, systemic signs are absent, though mild pleocytosis may occur. The cause is unknown, but the occurrence of the syndrome after vaccination or viral infection has led to the notion that it is an immunological or autoimmune response of some sort. Familial cases also occur with an autosomal dominant pattern.

467. The answer is c. (*Victor, p 1423.*) Familial dysautonomia, or Riley-Day disease, is an autosomal recessive disorder that affects primarily Jewish children. It is characterized by a small-fiber neuropathy affecting both myelinated and unmyelinated small fibers, thereby causing an impairment of pain and temperature sensation. Sympathetic and parasympathetic ganglia are also affected, causing the autonomic features. The autonomic manifestations may include loss of tears on crying, corneal ulceration, absence of pupillary reactivity, poor temperature regulation, excessive perspiration, abnormalities of blood pressure control, dysphagia, recurrent vomiting, and gastric and intestinal dilation. There is absence of the papillae of the tongue. There is no effective treatment other than symptomatic.

468. The answer is f. (*Victor, pp 1410–1413.*) Chronic inflammatory demyelinating polyneuropathy (CIDP) is similar to Guillain-Barré syndrome, but it takes a slowly progressive or remitting course rather than one of acute onset and rapid resolution. It is a polyradiculoneuropathy, implying that it affects the proximal portions of the nerves where they exit the spinal cord at the root level. This is the reason for the increase in protein, indicating an inflammatory disorder affecting nerve roots and causing demyelination. Because nerve roots are affected, this chronic neuropathy is not limited at onset to the distal feet, as a diabetic or other degenerative neuropathy might be. Patients therefore experience paresis and sensory loss proximally as well as distally.

469. The answer is g. (*Victor, pp 1389–1390.*) Porphyric polyneuropathy is associated with acute intermittent porphyria, which is a disorder of heme biosynthesis in the liver resulting from increased production and excretion of porphobilinogen and δ-aminolevulinic acid. The skin is not abnormal in this disorder. Instead, it is characterized by recurrent attacks of abdominal pain, gastroparesis and constipation (due to autonomic neuropathy), psychosis, axonal motor neuropathy, and autonomic instability. Seizures and syndrome of inappropriate antidiuretic hormone (SIADH) may also occur. Attacks may be fatal if respiratory paralysis or cardiac arrest occurs. Attacks may be provoked by porphyrinogenic drugs, such as barbiturates, phenytoin, sulfonamide antibiotics, and estrogens. These should be avoided in such patients. Treatment is best accomplished with use of intravenous hematin when supportive measures are not adequate or the case is severe.

470. The answer is f. (*Bradley, pp 2384–2385.*) Peripheral neuropathy from exposure to anesthetic agents is an occupational hazard faced by many health care providers. Megaloblastic anemia may develop along with peripheral neuropathy in nitrous oxide–induced neuropathy. This hazard is greatly increased if the health care worker uses the anesthetic agent as a recreational drug, which is a relatively common practice with nitrous oxide. Substance abuse involving agents intended for only occasional or short-term use, such as anesthetic agents, opiates, and opioids, must be rigorously explored with health professionals who develop inexplicable neurologic syndromes. Long-term abuse of nitrous oxide may lead to numbness, paresthesias, limb spasticity, and ataxia, signs pointing to central, rather than peripheral, nervous system damage. The syndrome is difficult to distinguish from vitamin B_{12} deficiency, and appears to result from interference with the vitamin B_{12}–dependent conversion of homocysteine to methionine.

471. The answer is b. (*Bradley, pp 1084–1086.*) Early in its evolution, sarcoid may be misconstrued as MS, especially if all the obvious deficits can be traced to the CNS. Optic atrophy and facial nerve palsies are common in sarcoid that gravitates to the nervous system. Peripheral neuropathy does not occur as a feature of MS, a strictly CNS disease, but it is still possible to have peripheral neuropathy along with MS, especially if the patient has been treated with a neurotoxic agent, such as cyclophosphamide.

472. The answer is c. *(Victor, pp 1212–1215.)* Thiamine deficiency commonly produces a painful sensory neuropathy in persons with alcoholism and poor nutrition. This man's history of esophageal varices and acknowledged alcohol abuse makes it highly likely that he has alcoholism-associated thiamine deficiency. Other vitamin deficiencies, including pyridoxine deficiency, are undoubtedly present, but thiamine deficiency is the most likely to evoke a painful neuropathy earliest. Dysesthesias and hyperpathia associated with this neuropathy may be so severe as to make it impossible for the patient to walk or tolerate any type of garment on the feet.

Neurological Emergencies

Questions

DIRECTIONS: Each item below contains a question followed by suggested responses. Select the **one best** response to each question.

473. A 55-year-old alcoholic man is brought in to the emergency room in a confused but nonagitated state. Significant exam findings include ophthalmoparesis, nystagmus, and ataxia. Emergency administration of which of the following medications is appropriate in the treatment of Wernicke's encephalopathy?

a. Glucose
b. Magnesium sulfate
c. Pyridoxine
d. Cyanocobalamin
e. Thiamine

474. A 66-year-old woman presents with weakness worsening over the past 3 hours. The weakness began in her face, but now involves most of her body. She had made her own jam several months before, and tasted a sample of it early this morning prior to discarding it because it smelled rancid. On further electrophysiologic testing, which of the following abnormalities would be most characteristic of this patient's illness?

a. Abnormal visual evoked responses (VERs)
b. Abnormal brainstem auditory evoked potentials
c. Posttetanic potentiation of the compound muscle action potential
d. Conduction block
e. Fibrillation potentials

475. A 6-month-old child is brought to the emergency room after having a generalized seizure at home. She is found to have a temperature of 102.5°F. Which of the following correctly reflects why this patient should be investigated with a spinal tap?

a.   All febrile seizures justify spinal taps
b.   Most febrile seizures are due to bacterial infections
c.   Febrile seizures cause increased intracranial pressure that must be relieved by withdrawing cerebrospinal fluid (CSF)
d.   Intrathecal antiepileptics must be given
e.   Children this age may have meningitis with no manifestations other than fever and seizures

476. A 17-year-old girl presents with subacute mental status change and left arm weakness. She had a viral illness 1 week ago, and now a diagnosis of acute disseminated encephalomyelitis (ADEM) is made. ADEM is a white matter disease that is distinguishable from multiple sclerosis (MS) by its being which of the following?

a.   Monophasic
b.   Rapidly lethal
c.   Associated with brainstem and spinal cord disease
d.   Associated with magnetic resonance imaging (MRI) lesions, which may resolve
e.   Associated with inflammatory changes in the brain

477. A 26-year-old woman with low back pain is seen in the clinic. She states that her pain began acutely, 2 weeks ago while lifting a couch. An MRI was performed in the ER and she was told that she has a "slipped disk" and sent home. The patient wants to know why surgery was not done immediately to correct the problem. Acute herniation of an intervertebral disk will require emergency surgery in which of the following circumstances?

a.   The disk is laterally herniated at C7
b.   The disk is causing radicular pain
c.   The cauda equina is being crushed
d.   A thoracic disk is involved
e.   The filum terminale is displaced

478. A 57-year-old man has been having nightly, unilateral, throbbing headaches. They have been occurring daily for the past week. The patient recalls having had a similar headache 5 years ago that lasted for several weeks. The patient has noticed that the headache is associated with lacrimation and a "stuffy nose." Ergot-amine prophylaxis has been partially successful. Which of the following is the most effective means of aborting this type of headache?

a. Inhaled 100% oxygen
b. Sublingual nitroglycerin
c. Oral methysergide
d. Oral propranolol
e. Dihydroergotamine suppository

479. A 32-year-old woman with alcoholism and cocaine use dating back at least 10 years comes to the emergency room after 48 h of recurrent vomiting and hematemesis. She reports abdominal discomfort that preceded the vomiting by a few days. For at least 36 h, she has been unable to keep ethanol in her stomach. Intravenous fluid replacement is started while she is being transported to the emergency room, and while in the emergency room she describes progressive blurring of vision. Over the course of 1 h, she becomes increasingly disoriented, ataxic, and dysarthric. Which of the following is the most likely explanation for her rapid deterioration?

a. Dehydration
b. Hypomagnesemia
c. Wernicke's encephalopathy
d. Hypoglycemia
e. Cocaine overdose

480. A 27-year-old man undergoes general anesthesia for a hernia repair. As the anesthesia begins, his jaw muscles tense and he becomes generally rigid. He becomes febrile, tachycardic, and tachypneic. Intravenous administration of which of the following agents may be lifesaving?

a. Suxamethonium
b. Nitrous oxide
c. Succinylcholine
d. Dantrolene
e. Phenobarbital

481. A 57-year-old woman with a history of diabetes mellitus and hyperthyroidism presents to the emergency room with a history of 2 days of vertical and horizontal diplopia. There is moderate orbital pain. On examination, her left eye is deviated downward and outward. It can be passively moved medially and upward. The pupils both react normally. Which of the following is the most likely etiology of her diplopia?

a. Hyperthyroidism
b. Diabetes mellitus
c. Cerebral aneurysm
d. Orbital pseudotumor
e. Orbital infection

482. A 33-year-old operating room nurse accidentally has blood splashed in her eyes during a procedure. The surgical resident who examines her immediately afterward notices that she has 2-mm anisocoria and sends her to the emergency room. She feels well, is alert and talkative, and has no motor dysfunction. On examination, the emergency room physician recognizes that the iris of the eye with the smaller pupil is pale blue, while that of the other eye is brown. Which of the following is the most likely etiology of the woman's anisocoria?

a. Conjunctivitis
b. Traumatic third-nerve palsy
c. Carotid artery dissection
d. Pupillary sphincter injury
e. Congenital

483. A 26-year-old man is brought into the emergency room after a motorcycle accident in which he was not wearing a helmet. Computed tomography (CT) scan shows bifrontal hemorrhagic contusions. The Glasgow Coma Scale (GCS) score is 6. He has no verbal response, opens his eyes to painful stimulation only, and shows a flexion response to pinch of the extremities. Which of the following is the most appropriate classification of this patient's head injury?

a. Minimal
b. Mild
c. Moderate
d. Severe
e. Vegetative

484. Two days following a motor vehicle accident, you are examining a 19-year-old right-handed man. He has a severe headache and "raccoon eyes." The presence of periorbital ecchymosis in a patient with traumatic head injury should be considered a sign of which of the following?

a. Subdural hemorrhage
b. Parenchymal hematoma
c. Ocular injury
d. Retinal detachment
e. Basilar skull fracture

485. Magnetic resonance imaging scan of a 19-year-old woman following a motor vehicle accident shows multiple foci of punctate hemorrhage. These are most likely indicative of which of the following?

a. Diffuse axonal injury (DAI)
b. Uncontrolled hypertension
c. Amyloid angiopathy
d. Ischemic infarction
e. Coagulopathy

486. Which of the following treatments should be recommended to improve the outcome of a patient with a traumatic head injury?

a. Corticosteroids
b. Prophylactic hyperventilation
c. Hyperthermia
d. Hypothermia
e. Prophylactic anticonvulsants

487. A 47-year-old woman begins to have difficulty swallowing food at dinner. Over the following 3 hours, she develops diplopia, dysarthria, and ultimately anarthria. She has a history of hypothyroidism and is on thyroid hormone replacement. There is no history of exposure to ticks or recent travel. On exam, she nods her head appropriately to questions, and she can write. Forced vital capacity is 500 mL, and she is intubated. She is afebrile, tachycardic, and normotensive. Bilateral ptosis and ophthalmoparesis are present; pupils are 6 mm in diameter and minimally reactive. Facial sensation is intact. Bifacial paresis is present, and the tongue is weak. Extremity muscle bulk and tone are normal, and proximal strength is 4/5 in her arms and legs. Finger and toe movements are rapid and symmetric. Plantar responses are flexor. Blood tests are normal. Motor nerve conduction studies show low-amplitude compound muscle action potentials with normal velocities. Sensory nerve action potentials are normal. Which of the following organisms is most likely be responsible for this woman's syndrome?

a. Cytomegalovirus (CMV)
b. *Treponema pallidum*
c. *Chlamydia pneumoniae*
d. *Clostridium botulinum*
e. *Campylobacter jejuni*

488. A 66-year-old woman presents with fever and a generalized convulsion. Neuroimaging and lumbar puncture are most consistent with a diagnosis of herpes encephalitis. Which of the following is the most appropriate treatment for this patient?

a. Decadron
b. Amphotericin B
c. Gamma globulin
d. Methotrexate
e. Acyclovir

489. A 41-year-old right-handed woman has had one day of progressive weakness. The symptoms began in her extraocular muscles and then spread quickly to involve other muscles in her face before her entire body felt weak. The history is significant for the recent ingestion of home-canned fruit. The underlying mechanism of botulism is which of the following?

a. Antibodies to the acetylcholine receptor
b. Antibodies to the calcium receptor
c. Depolarizing blockade of the potassium channel
d. Impaired formation of acetylcholine-laden vesicles
e. Toxic muscle necrosis
f. Demyelination

490. A 22-year-old woman presents to the emergency room with an episode of acute painful loss of vision in the right eye. On examination, there is a right afferent pupillary defect and papillitis on funduscopic examination. She has no history of neurologic symptoms. An MRI shows a few foci of T2 signal increase in a periventricular distribution. Which of the following is the most appropriate treatment for presumed optic neuritis in this patient?

a. Oral prednisone
b. Intravenous methylprednisolone
c. Cyclophosphamide
d. Plasma exchange
e. Intravenous gamma globulin

491. A previously healthy 23-year-old woman has had 2 weeks of blurry vision in her left eye. Multiple tests, including visual evoked potentials, are performed. The diagnosis of optic neuritis is made. What is the approximate likelihood that this patient will eventually develop multiple sclerosis?

a. 0%
b. 5%
c. 25%
d. 40%
e. 75%

492. A 27-year-old man who 6 months ago had optic neuritis presents to the emergency room describing a brief, sharp pain radiating into the left side of his face. The vision in his eye has largely recovered, and there is no evidence of sensory loss on the right side of his face. He describes the pain as ice pick–like and grimaces with each attack. He is most likely to have symptomatic relief from his facial pain if he is managed with which of the following drugs?

a. Aspirin
b. Acetaminophen
c. Ibuprofen
d. Carbamazepine
e. Codeine

493. A patient who has been diagnosed with multiple sclerosis has had recurrent episodes of bed wetting (enuresis) over the preceding month. This should decrease with the administration of which of the following drugs?

a. Imipramine
b. Phenytoin
c. Carbamazepine
d. Baclofen
e. Methacholine

494. Over the course of a few months, a patient with multiple sclerosis develops painful spasticity in her left leg that interferes with extension of her leg. The spasticity progresses to the point of interfering with her sleep. Which of the following is the most appropriate treatment for this patient?

a. Imipramine
b. Phenytoin
c. Carbamazepine
d. Baclofen
e. Methacholine

495. A 47-year-old man arrives at the emergency room in a coma. His wife reports that he developed shaking movements and abnormal breathing sounds in the middle of the night. His shaking and the sounds woke her, but she was unable to wake him. He has been somewhat forgetful over the prior 3 months, but has seemed well otherwise. Examination in the emergency room reveals an unresponsive man who exhibits generalized convulsions every 10 min. He is afebrile and incontinent of urine. The physician on call believes the patient is in status epilepticus, and should consequently immediately order which of the following?

a. An intraventricular drain to monitor intracranial pressure
b. Lorazepam (Ativan) for intravenous administration
c. Carbamazepine (Tegretol) by nasogastric tube
d. Phenytoin (Dilantin) by nasogastric tube
e. Gabapentin (Neurontin) by nasogastric tube

496. During the initial treatment of a patient with status epilepticus, a nurse reports that the patient has just lost bladder control and that the urine appears darker than normal. The responsible physician examines the bedsheets and agrees with the nurse's assessment. The physician should immediately institute which measure?

a. Order placement of an indwelling urinary catheter
b. Order methacholine to regulate bladder emptying
c. Request a surgical consultation in anticipation of an exploratory laparotomy
d. Order placement of a condom catheter
e. Request a urologic consultation to assess the incontinence

497. A 64-year-old man presents to the emergency room with convulsive seizures. A precontrast CT of the brain reveals a hemorrhagic mass in the left frontal lobe, but there is little apparent shift of brain structures and no ventricular enlargement. Two hours after the patient's seizures have stopped, his blood pressure is still elevated at 180/100 mmHg and his pulse is slow at 50/min. Although the patient is still unconscious, he appears to have decreased tone on the right side of his body. The physician should request which of the following interventions?

a. Intravenous clonidine (Catapres) to lower the blood pressure
b. Placement of a cardiac pacemaker to manage the bradyarrhythmia
c. Neurosurgical consult
d. Placement of a ventriculoperitoneal shunt
e. Intravenous tissue plasminogen activator (TPA)

498. A 52-year-old woman presented to the emergency room with a new onset aphasia. A hemorrhagic left frontal mass is apparent on head CT. The neurosurgical consultant decides to explore the site of the hemorrhage and evacuate the mass that has collected there. He sends tissue from the margin of the blood clot for a frozen section analysis by the pathologist. The tissue is felt to be Kernohan grade IV astrocytoma. Which of the following post-operative therapies is most reasonable?

a. Cranial radiotherapy
b. Intravenous methotrexate
c. Intravenous fludarabine
d. Intravenous cyclophosphamide
e. Intravenous daunorubicin

499. A 56-year-old man is brought into the emergency room after having collapsed at work 30 minutes ago. He has no medical history and takes no medications. He is alert and speaking but has no awareness of any deficit. He has a right gaze deviation, dense left face and arm plegia, and mild left leg weakness. When asked to raise his legs, he lifts only the right leg. He has reduced blink to threat from the left side. Which of the following is the most appropriate initial diagnostic step?

a. Head CT
b. Cerebral angiogram
c. C-spine MRI
d. T2-weighted brain MRI
e. Skull x-rays

500. A 63-year-old man presents to the emergency room with a right hemi-paresis and nonfluent aphasia that began acutely 45 minutes ago. Blood pressure is 160/80, coagulation studies are normal, and there is no recent history of bleeding. A head CT scan shows no evidence of intracranial hemorrhage. Which of the following is the most appropriate therapy at this point?

a. Intravenous rTPA
b. Intravenous streptokinase
c. Oral aspirin
d. Intravenous heparin
e. Intravenous mannitol

Neurological Emergencies

Answers

473. The answer is e. (*Victor, pp 1206–1212.*) Without rapid replacement of thiamine stores, the patient with acute Wernicke's encephalopathy may die. Usually 50 to 100 mg of thiamine is given intravenously immediately. This is followed over the course of a few days with supplementary thiamine injections of 50 to 100 mg. Without thiamine, the patient will develop periaqueductal and mamillary body lesions, which will be clinically apparent as autonomic failure. With chronic thiamine deficiency, neuronal loss occurs in alcoholic persons at least partly because of this relative vitamin deficiency. Purkinje and other cells in the cerebellar vermis will be lost to so dramatic an extent that gross atrophy of the superior cerebellar vermis will be evident.

474. The answer is c. (*Victor, pp 286–287.*) Botulism is a disorder of the neuromuscular junction (NMJ). The characteristic findings are decremental response of the muscles to repetitive stimulation of the nerve at a low frequency (2 to 5 Hz) and incremental response to repetitive stimulation at high frequency (20 to 50 Hz). Other disorders of the NMJ, such as myasthenia gravis and Lambert-Eaton myasthenic syndrome (LEMS), also manifest with decremental response to repetitive stimulation at low frequencies due to depletion of acetylcholine in the synaptic cleft. Higher rates of stimulation lead to increased calcium in the presynaptic terminal, which allows more acetylcholine to be released in presynaptic disorders such as botulism and LEMS, thereby increasing the response of muscle. However, in myasthenia gravis, which is characterized by loss of acetylcholine receptors postsynaptically, there is no increase in response at higher rates of stimulation, because there is already a maximal amount of acetylcholine present in the synaptic cleft. Abnormal visual evoked and brainstem auditory evoked potentials would be seen in disorders affecting central pathways, such as MS. Conduction block occurs in demyelinating disorders affecting the nerves. Fibrillation potentials are present in denervation and certain myopathic conditions; they may occur in botulism, as well as in patients treated with botulinum toxin for therapeutic purposes, but this is not diagnostic of clinical botulism.

475. The answer is e. *(Swaiman, p 677.)* Between birth and 1 year of age, what appears to be a simple febrile seizure may actually be a seizure provoked by a bacterial meningitis. The agents most likely to be responsible in a 6-month-old child are *Haemophilus influenzae, Streptococcus pneumoniae,* and *Neisseria meningitidis.* Since the introduction of vaccination against *H. influenzae,* however, the incidence of meningitis due to this organism has been drastically reduced. Below 3 months of age, group B streptococci, *Escherichia coli,* and *Listeria monocytogenes* must also be considered. All require rapid diagnosis and early treatment if the child is to survive. Even though the child may not have substantial neck stiffness, the CSF will typically reveal a glucose content less than two-thirds the serum level, elevated WBC count, and increased protein content. The responsible organism may be isolated and cultured, but treatment of the meningitis should begin before the organism is identified. A delay of hours in treatment may be lethal. Intravenous antibiotics should be started as soon as there is convincing evidence that febrile seizures are secondary to a bacterial meningitis. The drug chosen should be the one most effective against the most probable organism. The child's age, exposure, and symptomatology must all be considered in deciding what organism is most likely responsible for the infection.

476. The answer is a. *(Bradley, pp 1659–1662.)* Acute disseminated encephalomyelitis is a demyelinating disease of the brain, brainstem, and spinal cord that is indistinguishable from MS on MRI. It is, however, monophasic, meaning that it occurs acutely on a single occasion and not in a recurrent fashion like MS. It usually develops within days or weeks of a viral illness or an immunization. Childhood exanthems are especially likely to precipitate ADEM, as are smallpox and rabies immunizations. As in MS, the lesions associated with ADEM usually produce perivenous demyelination with sparing of the nerve axons.

477. The answer is c. *(Victor, p 217.)* Surgery may eventually be necessary with any intervertebral disk herniation, but with acute, massive cauda equina injury, surgery must be performed before the deficits are irreversible. Signs of cauda equina compression include loss of bladder and bowel control and paraparesis or paraplegia. An acutely evolving focal motor deficit in the legs, such as a footdrop, associated with sphincter dysfunction is justification for emergency laminectomy and disk resection. Preoperative studies should be obtained to be sure that the responsible lesion is disk herniation, because metastatic cancers, such as prostate and breast carcinoma, may imitate acute disk herniations. Establishing the identity of the lesion is important because many tumors are better managed with high-dose corticosteroids and radiation therapy than with surgery. Osteomyelitis of the vertebral body may also produce cauda equina compression; a decompressive laminectomy is usually indicated with focal infections of this sort to maximize the recovery achieved with antibiotic therapy.

478. The answer is a. *(Victor, p 191.)* Oxygen may terminate a cluster headache within minutes. Some physicians recommend inhaling 4 L/min of 100% oxygen by mask as soon as signs of an impending headache develop. This has prompted many sufferers of cluster headaches to keep a cylinder of compressed oxygen at home during the season when they are most likely to develop such headaches. Cluster headaches usually occur at night when the patient is asleep, and so practical access to the oxygen tank is possible. Methysergide is effective in preventing cluster headaches for many persons, but it does rarely cause the worrisome adverse effect of fibrosis. Retroperitoneal, pulmonary, and endocardial fibroses are potential adverse effects of methysergide. Sublingual nitroglycerin may in fact trigger a headache and is not recommended for patients with migraine or cluster headaches. Propranolol is a β-adrenergic blocking agent that is useful in the prophylaxis of some vascular headaches, but it is of no value in aborting a cluster headache. Dihydroergotamine suppositories may abort some vascular headaches, but they do not have as obvious an effect in cluster as in classic or common migraine syndromes.

479. The answer is c. *(Victor, pp 1206–1212.)* Wernicke's encephalopathy is a potentially fatal consequence of thiamine deficiency, a problem for which this woman was at risk by virtue of being an alcoholic. When she came to the emergency room, intravenous fluids were started that probably contained glucose. The stress of a large glucose load will abruptly deplete the CNS of the little thiamine it has available and will precipitate the sort of deterioration evident in this woman. Features characteristic of a Wernicke's encephalopathy include deteriorating level of consciousness, autonomic disturbances, ocular motor problems, and gait difficulty. Autonomic disturbances may include lethal hypotension or profound hypothermia. Hemorrhagic necrosis in periventricular gray matter will be evident in this woman's brain if she dies. The mamillary bodies are especially likely to be extensively damaged.

480. The answer is d. (*Victor, p 1563.*) Malignant hyperthermia is characterized by acute severe fever, tachypnea, tachycardia, and rigidity, and high mortality rate if left untreated. It is typically precipitated by volatile anesthetics, especially halothane, or muscle relaxants such as succinylcholine. Patients may become severely acidotic and develop rhabdomyolysis. Pathology shows diffuse segmental muscle necrosis. It appears to be a metabolic myopathy in which there is abnormal release of calcium from the sarcoplasmic reticulum (SR) and ineffectual uptake afterward. Genetic defects in the ryanodine receptor, involved in calcium flux in the SR, are responsible for about 10% of cases, although as yet unidentified abnormalities of this or related proteins probably play a role in most cases. It is inherited in an autosomal dominant fashion. Certain other myopathies, including Duchenne muscular dystrophy and central core myopathy, are associated with this condition as well. Treatment consists of discontinuation of anesthesia, administration of dantrolene, which prevents release of calcium from the SR, and supportive measures.

481. The answer is b. (*Victor, pp 286–287.*) The third cranial nerve (the oculomotor nerve) controls several movements of the globe, including upward and medial movements, through its control of the medial rectus, superior rectus, and inferior oblique muscles. Its inactivity leads to displacement of the eye down and out. Fourth-nerve palsy leads to weakness of the superior oblique muscle, with resultant difficulty looking down and medially; patients often complain of trouble walking down stairs. Sixth-nerve palsy produces weakness of the lateral rectus muscle, causing horizontal diplopia. Fractures of the orbit can entrap individual muscles, but there is no history of this here. Thyroid ophthalmopathy, or Graves' disease, can produce diplopia, but there is usually proptosis or lid retraction. The inferior and medial recti are most frequently affected. Because this is caused by infiltration of the muscles, there is usually limitation of passive movement of the eyes (i.e., forced ductions). Diabetes is a common cause of third-nerve palsy (approximately 10% of cases). Usually, when diabetes is the cause, there is sparing of the pupillomotor parasympathetic fibers, which travel on the outside of the nerve. Diabetes causes third-nerve palsy via nerve infarction, which affects the interior of the nerve but spares the external fibers. Compressive lesions, however, can injure the surface fibers, thereby causing pupillary dilation due to unopposed sympathetic activity.

482. The answer is e. *(Victor, p 296.)* Sympathetic innervation of the iris is required for the change in the color of the iris to occur after birth and infancy. Congenital Horner syndrome, which may be inherited as an autosomal dominant trait, is characterized by failure of one eye to develop normal iris color (heterochromia iridis). Any injury to the eye after this early developmental period would not be expected to leave a difference in eye color from one side to the other.

483. The answer is d. *(Bradley, pp 1134–1135.)* The GCS was introduced in 1974 by Teasdale and Jennett. It has three parts: best motor response (1 to 6 points), best verbal response (1 to 5 points), and eye opening (1 to 4 points). The total score ranges from 3 to 15 (normal). The presence of coma is defined as GCS of 8 or less, which represents a patient who does not follow commands, speak, or open the eyes. Head injuries may be defined on the basis of the GCS: mild injury (GCS 14 to 15), moderate injury (GCS 9 to 13), and severe injury (GCS ≤ 8). Although patients with mild head injuries may receive a score of 15, the maximum on the GCS, they may still have more subtle cognitive difficulties that are not reflected by this easy-to-use and simple scale.

484. The answer is e. *(Bradley, p 49.)* The presence of periorbital ecchymosis (raccoon eyes), ecchymosis over the mastoid region (Battle's sign), hemotympanum (blood behind the eardrum), or CSF rhinorrhea or otorrhea should be considered evidence of a basilar skull fracture.

485. The answer is a. *(Bradley, pp 1129–1130.)* Diffuse axonal injury is the most common cause of coma in the head-injured patient without an intracranial mass lesion. It is characterized pathologically by diffusely spread axonal swellings affecting the white matter, corpus callosum, and upper brainstem. These foci are usually hemorrhagic. The etiology is thought to be due to shearing forces on axons in certain susceptible regions of the brain, notably those that are particularly vulnerable to rotational forces, such as the subcortical white matter, corpus callosum, and upper brainstem. Uncontrolled hypertension may occur in patients with hypertension, but would be unlikely to produce this pattern of injury. Amyloid angiopathy causes multiple hemorrhages, but affects elderly patients. The decreased cerebral perfusion pressure associated with brain swelling and increased intracranial pressure could cause ischemic infarction, but this would not be expected to give this appearance on MRI. Coagulopathies also occur in up to 20% of patients.

486. The answer is d. (*Bradley, pp 1123–1124.*) Hypothermia has been shown to reduce cerebral injury from ischemia both in experimental models and in clinical studies of patients with traumatic brain injury. Hypothermia decreases cerebral metabolism, reduces acidosis, attenuates changes in the blood-brain barrier, and inhibits the release of excitatory neurotransmitters that can be harmful. Corticosteroids, prophylactic hyperventilation, and prophylactic anticonvulsants have not been shown to be of benefit in the long-term prognosis of severely head-injured patients. Hyperthermia is detrimental to such patients.

487. The answer is d. (*Victor, pp 1274–1275.*) The rapid onset of bulbar paresis is consistent with acute inflammatory demyelinating polyneuropathy (AIDP, or Guillain-Barré syndrome), botulism, tick paralysis, and several other conditions. The normal conduction velocities argue against demyelinating neuropathy, which may be associated with *C. jejuni*. Cytomegalovirus and *T. pallidum* may cause several different neurologic syndromes, but acute bulbar paresis is not among them. *C. pneumoniae* is under investigation as a cause of atherosclerosis, strokes, and MS, but it does not cause acute motor weakness.

488. The answer is e. (*Victor, pp 794–795.*) The diagnosis of herpes encephalitis is more controversial than the treatment. Many authorities believe brain biopsy should be performed whenever the diagnosis is suspected, but the availability of polymerase chain reaction (PCR) for herpes simplex virus (HSV) in the CSF and MRI have made diagnosis easier. In the appropriate clinical setting, these tests may obviate the need for brain biopsy, although it still remains the definitive test. A high index of suspicion must be maintained and treatment must be initiated quickly. Acyclovir must be given intravenously for 10 days.

489. The answer is d. *(Victor, pp 286–287.)* Botulinum toxin, a 150-kDa polypeptide chain, is cleaved into two chains: a 100-kDa chain required for neuronal binding and a 50-kDa chain that destroys important proteins required for neurotransmitter packaging. The toxin reduces the amount of acetylcholine available for release when a motor neuron is depolarized. Eight serotypes of botulism toxin are now recognized: A, B, C1, C2, D, E, F, and G. Although the toxins cleave different proteins, they interfere with the same step in vesicle formation.

490. The answer is b. *(Bradley, pp 1639, 1647.)* Clinical trials have shown that intravenous methylprednisolone for an attack of optic neuritis reduces the likelihood of developing MS over 2 years from 16.7% to 7.5%. It also is associated with a better outcome than oral prednisone. Intravenous methylprednisolone is thus recommended by most experts as appropriate therapy for acute exacerbations of MS involving more than sensory manifestations alone.

491. The answer is e. *(Victor, pp 962–963.)* The risk of developing MS after optic neuritis was 74% in women and 34% in men after 15 years of follow-up in one study. Other studies have found similarly high rates. The longer the follow-up period, and the more rigorously signs of MS are sought, the more likely it is that MS will be found. Most patients develop the MS within 5 years of the initial attack of optic neuritis. Magnetic resonance imaging scanning of the brain at the time of optic neuritis is, in fact, abnormal in between 50% and 72% of patients, suggesting the presence of subclinical MS.

492. The answer is d. *(Victor, pp 196–198.)* This man has exhibited two different complaints separated in time and space, a clinical pattern that must raise the possibility of MS in a man this age. The pattern of pain is suggestive of trigeminal neuralgia (tic douloureux), an idiopathic facial pain syndrome that often develops in persons with MS. Alternatives to carbamazepine in the palliation of trigeminal neuralgia include phenytoin and baclofen.

493. The answer is a. *(Bradley, p 1655.)* Bladder dysfunction with MS is usually a consequence of corticospinal tract disease. This lesion of the upper motor neuron produces a spastic bladder. Tricyclic antidepressants such as imipramine exert an anticholinergic effect and thereby inhibit premature emptying of the bladder. Cholinergic drugs, such as methacholine, are useful if the patient has a flaccid bladder, but that is much less frequently the problem with MS.

494. The answer is d. (*Bradley, p 1654.*) Baclofen affects spasticity through an unknown mechanism and may cause considerable sedation. Sedation is less a concern if spasticity is interfering with the patient's ability to sleep. The drug is usually given orally at a dose of 10 mg three or four times daily, but most patients must start at a much lower dose and gradually build up tolerance. Baclofen has been given intrathecally with an implanted pump injector, but this highly invasive therapy is appropriate only in patients with extreme spasticity. Candidates for intrathecal treatment are functionally paraplegic and may recover considerable mobility with elimination of the spasticity. Tizanidine is a centrally active α_2-adrenergic agonist that appears to relieve spasticity without affecting strength.

495. The answer is b. (*Victor, pp 361–362.*) There are several different options in initiating the treatment of status epilepticus. Some clinicians recommend intravenous diazepam (Valium) as the initial medication, but this has a short-lived effect. Lorazepam (Ativan) is equally effective and has a more persistent effect. Phenytoin should be used in conjunction with a benzodiazepine to prevent relapse after the benzodiazepine's effect abates, but it must be administered parenterally in the setting of status in order to achieve rapid therapeutic levels. Although phenytoin cannot be given at more than 50 mg/min because of the risk of cardiac depression associated with more rapid infusion rates, the more recently available fosphenytoin can be administered intramuscularly or intravenously at rates up to 150 mg/min. Carbamazepine (Tegretol) and gabapentin (Neurontin) are not available as intravenous medications, and their absorption from the gastrointestinal tract is unacceptably slow for the treatment of status epilepticus. Intracranial pressure (ICP) will usually be increased during status epilepticus, but that is of no immediate clinical consequence, and monitoring of the ICP in status epilepticus is inappropriate in the absence of a specific indication such as documented head trauma or other mass lesion. Intracranial pressure is routinely monitored by neurosurgeons in cases of severe head trauma to provide early warning of catastrophic changes within the head.

496. The answer is d. (*Victor, pp 286–287.*) Urinary incontinence is an expected consequence of status epilepticus and consequently should not arouse concern for abdominal or urologic disturbances. Keeping the patient dry is important because of the risk of skin breakdown with any comatose patient, but mechanical intervention is sufficient. An indwelling catheter is unnecessary and introduces the risk of urinary tract infection. A condom catheter will keep the patient dry, allow urine to be collected, and enable the staff to more rigorously monitor fluid output. The urine is likely to be darkened by myoglobin, a pigment that collects in the urine when muscle breaks down after protracted seizure activity.

497. The answer is c. (*Victor, pp 901–903.*) An expanding intracranial mass will produce an elevated blood pressure and a slow heart rate. This is called the *Cushing effect.* This man may have a neoplasm in the brain or amyloid bleed. The site of the hemorrhage is unlikely with chronic hypertension or aneurysm. A biopsy of the mass would help identify the underlying lesion, although it is not urgent. Metastatic neoplastic disease is a possibility but is less likely than a glioblastoma multiforme at this age. The administration of TPA is contraindicated because this drug will increase the risk of rebleeding. Placement of a drain is not suggested by the clinical picture because there was no evidence of obstruction to the flow of CSF.

498. The answer is a. (*Bradley, p 1432.*) There are several different grading schemes for astrocytoma, but Kernohan's classification of grades from I (least malignant) to IV (most malignant) is the one most widely used. Glioblastoma multiforme is an older term for the grade IV astrocytoma and is still in general use. This is a highly malignant tumor that develops most often in the cerebral hemispheres. The most malignant tumors usually exhibit areas of necrosis and have a poor prognosis. Survival with glioblastoma multiforme is usually measured in months rather than years. Treatment generally consists of gross total resection and radiation therapy. Survival may be increased to 40 weeks after this combination of therapies, whereas it is on average only 14 weeks after surgery alone. The intravenous medications listed are antineoplastic agents, but they are not effective against this type of tumor. The only chemotherapy generally regarded as useful for this type of primary brain tumor is 1,3-bis (2-chloroethyl)-1-nitrosourea (BCNU), which increases survival only marginally.

499. The answer is a. *(Bradley, pp 1236–1238.)* The head CT scan is the mainstay of emergency department diagnosis of acute stroke. It is crucial to exclude intracranial hemorrhage prior to the potential administration of intravenous thrombolytic agents. A cerebral angiogram may play a role in the management of the acute stroke patient, particularly if there is evidence of cerebral or subarachnoid hemorrhage, or if there exists a possibility of performing intra-arterial thrombolysis, but CT scan is required first. T2-weighted MRI may also show ischemic and hemorrhagic injury, but infarction may not appear this quickly on MRI and hemorrhage may also be missed. MRI is also not as widely available as CT. In the absence of evidence of trauma at the time of the patient's fall, C-spine MRI and skull x-rays play no role in management.

500. The answer is a. *(Bradley, pp 1236–1238.)* In a large, multicenter randomized trial sponsored by the NIH, thrombolytic therapy with intravenous rTPA has been shown to be of benefit to patients with acute ischemic stroke who can be treated early enough. The study demonstrated a statistically significant benefit for the use of rTPA in the treatment of ischemic stroke patients who can be treated within 3 h of symptom onset. A total of 624 patients arriving at the hospital within 3 h of symptom onset underwent CT scan to exclude hemorrhagic stroke. Patients were randomized to receive either 0.9 mg/kg of rTPA or placebo. At 3 months, treated patients were at least 30% more likely to have minimal or no disability on several disability scales. Even with a symptomatic hemorrhage rate of 6.4% within 36 hours among the active treatment patients, the mortality and disability among treated patients was less than that among placebo patients at 3 months. The overall acute neurologic deterioration even after accounting for early hemorrhages was the same in treated and placebo patients, indicating that the increased risk of hemorrhage with rTPA therapy is offset by an increased risk of neurologic deterioration from progressing stroke, cerebral edema, and other causes in nontreated patients. The benefit of rTPA was not limited to patients with cardioembolic or large-vessel strokes, but also benefited patients with small-vessel strokes, who had a better prognosis.

Bibliography

Bradley W, et al (eds): *Neurology in Clinical Practice*, 4/e. Boston, Butterworth-Heinemann, 2004.

DeMyer WE: *Technique of the Neurologic Examination A Programmed Text*, 5/e. New York, McGraw-Hill, 2004.

Greenberg JO (ed): *Neuroimaging*, 2/e. New York, McGraw-Hill, 1999.

Kandel ER, et al (eds): *Principles of Neural Science*, 4/e. New York, McGraw-Hill, 2000.

Kasper DL, et al (eds): *Harrison's Principles of Internal Medicine*, 16/e. New York, McGraw-Hill, 2005.

Lee SH, et al (eds): *Cranial MRI and CT*, 4/e. New York, McGraw-Hill, 1999.

Patten J: *Neurological Differential Diagnosis*, 2/e. London, Springer-Verlag, 2001.

Swaiman K, Ashwal S (eds): *Pediatric Neurology Principles and Practice*, 3/e. St. Louis, Mosby, 1999.

Victor M, et al: *Principles of Neurology*, 7/e. New York, McGraw-Hill, 2001.

Watts RL and Koller WC (eds): *Movement Disorders Neurologic Principles and Practice*, 2/e. New York, McGraw-Hill, 2004.

Index